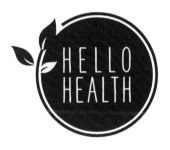

HELLO, HEALTH

Navigating and Winning Better Cognitive and Immune Function

A Guidebook for Saving
21st Century Families

PAMELA WIRTH

Melanie Alarcio, M.D., & Jeremy Appleton, N.D.

ISBN: 978-1-7331535-0-8 (paperback)
ISBN: 978-1-7331535-1-5 (ebook)
Library of Congress Control Number: 2019912455

Published by Hello Health Nutrition LLC
Email: support@hellohealthnutrition.com

Book Design by Jill Ronsley, Sun Editing & Book Design, suneditwrite.com

10 9 8 7 6 5 4 3 2 1

Printed and bound in the USA

CONTENTS

FOREWORD

I'VE KNOWN PAM FOR ALMOST 25 years. We met when we both did a college study abroad program in London in 1995, and now see each other about once a year even though we live in different states. We've gotten better about it now that our kids are older, and just enjoyed a girls' weekend here in Austin, Texas. I shared with Pam my concerns about my son's health.

My son is ten and was diagnosed with ADD, anxiety, and severe OCD (an offshoot of the anxiety). It all started when he was born. There was always something different about him compared to my other two—just the way he seemed to process things. He didn't have the same temperament.

At age five, he got the flu over Christmas break. Jack was in preschool at the time, and in January his teacher called me and said he was panicked inside the classroom. He developed severe claustrophobia after that. He wouldn't go inside our small church, he wouldn't go in the classroom, and he wouldn't get in the car unless you were in the car first, which was hard to do.

We went to a psychiatrist at the time and they gave us Zoloft. He's been on it ever since. We've gone to different doctors, trying to find the right medication. Now, they've increased his dose of Zoloft since his anxiety and OCD have seemed to worsen. He's also on a stimulant during the school year because he's struggling in school (we still haven't found the right stimulant for him). He just can't focus. We've done a battery of tests to make sure there is no learning disability but have not found one. He has perplexed us because he's had high testing scores but still can't complete multi-step math problems. He just can't sit down and focus. It's really sad and we're at a loss regarding what to do next. We've tried to change his diet, we've seen several different doctors, we've tried cognitive therapy, and we haven't found the magic combination yet.

I shared all of this with Pam, and it was like a whole new world opened up.

I've looked at this from a traditional approach—you go to a psychiatrist, you get a medication, maybe you go to therapy, you change your diet. But talking to Pam was like an *aha!* moment. All the light bulbs turned on. It seemed like what she had gone through in her family, health-wise, was very similar to what we are facing today in ours.

When Pam talked about all she had learned, it just started making sense: the immune system response, the MTHFR gene, vitamin deficiencies, and everything she's learned about testing for Strep titers, Epstein-Barr virus, mycoplasma, Lyme, and CMV. She said that she had been a Strep carrier, and how it caused major problems. She shared what she knew about the genetic component of neurological and autoimmune diseases. This resonated with me as my father had issues, so there is definitely a genetic component to what we've been dealing with.

Pam gave me information about how to take a functional medicine approach to the kinds of symptoms my son is experiencing—something you'll learn about throughout this book—which was extremely exciting to hear about.

Our conversations put me on new course of thinking. We keep spending thousands of dollars going to all these experts, and we keep getting new prescriptions with new side effects, and we lose more time in school. We are in this vicious cycle, and it's time for a different approach.

To hear Pam's story, to find out that she's taking charge, and to learn of the way she advocated for her son...it inspired me to ask the right questions. To do more research. To not just leave it to the so-called experts to decide what needs to be done. After I talked to Pam, I went to a Health Coach and learned more about potential nutrient deficiencies. We are going to have her test my son to see what changes we can make there. She referred us to a doctor here in town, a former ENT surgeon who now focuses as a Neuro-Immune Specialist. Unfortunately, the earliest we can get into see him is six months from now.

One thing I love about Pam's approach is looking at the health of the entire family. It's not just our son; he's part of a larger genetic whole. The more we find out about myself, my husband, and our extended family, the more tools and ideas we will have.

I am so excited and so appreciative that Pam wrote this book. I think it's going to help a lot of people get on a better path.

—Danika Melia

INTRODUCTION

OUR MINDS AND BODIES ARE one: two parts of the same whole. They are not two distinct entities. What you put into your body affects your mind, and when your body gets sick, your mental health and behavior can change. It sounds so obvious, doesn't it? It's almost like saying the sky is blue. Unfortunately, medical science has long treated our minds and bodies separately. There are separate drugs, separate doctors, separate treatments.

It's time to change our thinking.

My family learned this firsthand, and I'm hoping our story can help to change the dialogue on how we can keep our children and families healthy, whether the issue you're facing is an autoimmune disorder, a diagnosis of Type 1 diabetes, autism spectrum disorder, anxiety, depression, or a whole host of other diseases.

If you've picked up this book, you know how quickly your child's health can change. It's terrifying. One minute, your world is in order. The next, everything has fallen apart and even the doctors are stumped.

My story began the first week of January many years ago, when our son Ryan (not his real name), who was turning six that year, had a terrible illness and sinus infection. It was so severe, in fact, that we had to cancel his birthday party. What we didn't know then but do know now is that he was suffering from an antibiotic-resistant strain of Streptococcus, Epstein-Barr virus, and Cytomegalovirus infections simultaneously, which sparked autoimmune encephalitis. This cascade of illness caused Ryan to developmentally regress by several years in what seemed like a single night.

Before this all happened, our son was "a smiley, happy, care-free, silly child who is intensively active in school, sports and home. He has a wild sense of humor and loves people." Those were the words we used to describe how Ryan came across to other people. This was what we were used to—until he got so sick.

That's when the light went out of our son's eyes. Ryan began experiencing severe headaches. He began speaking in baby talk and made loud nonsensical sounds. He had constantly dilated pupils and blinking eyes; he began twirling around, sucking his thumb and acting uncharacteristically clingy. One night he even reverted to crawling. This was all within a matter of 2-3 weeks, which made it very difficult to react, let alone understand.

Brain Under Attack

Despite these sudden and highly alarming symptoms, visits to a number of conventional medical practitioners led to un-acceptable recommendations ranging from antidepressants to a portal shunt for immunoglobulin therapy. We were offered very little in the way of diagnostic options and in more than one instance, were dismissed with the assurance that kids will be kids!

Our story was highlighted in Beth Lambert's 2018 book *Brain Under Attack*. As a result of the interest it garnered, I was inspired to delve a little deeper and provide practical tools and approaches for families struggling with similar challenges.

My goal is to give families a new understanding of how certain illnesses can trigger a neurological response—and what to do about it.

Lambert is an inspiration and her work is a good resource for families. She is the Founder and Executive Director of Epidemic Answers, a 501(c)(3) non-profit organization dedicated to educating the public about the epidemic of chronic illness affecting our youth, and helping parents find healing solutions. I encourage you to visit and donate if you are able.

A Growing Medical Crisis

Our family is not alone in coming face to face with this kind of terrifying health scare. According to the Sarkie Mazmanian Lab at Caltech University in Pasadena, California, the Western world is experiencing a growing medical crisis. There has been a significant increase in instances of immune disorders such as inflammatory bowel disease, celiac disease, rheumatoid arthritis, Crohn's disease, asthma, Type 1 diabetes, multiple sclerosis, and autism.[1]

Until quite recently, scientists and clinicians rarely recognized a link between gut health, environmental and infectious

---

1 "We All Live In A Microbial World" sarkis.caltech.edu Accessed April 2, 2019.

triggers, autoimmune disease, and neurological symptoms such as anxiety and depression.

Today, that's changing.

Fortunately, more and more doctors are recognizing the intrinsic relationship between systemic, infectious, and autoimmune disease and neurological symptoms—both in pediatric and adult populations. In conjunction with advances in diagnostic techniques, this awareness is leading to the identification of root cause and targeted treatment protocols. Locating these progressive practitioners can be a challenge, however.

What is Autoimmune Disease?

According to the National Institute of Environmental Health Sciences (NIEHS), autoimmune diseases result from a dysfunction of the immune system, which is supposed to protect us from disease and infection. When the immune system begins producing antibodies that attack healthy cells inside of us, an individual is said to have an autoimmune disease. These diseases can affect any part of the body, including the brain, leading to emotional, cognitive, and developmental disorders.

Autoantibodies are the hallmark of autoimmune diseases, but the issues affecting the brain are more commonly caused by inflammation, which is also a function of the immune system. Toxins can also play a role. These are often related to intestinal hyperpermeability, or leaky gut—something you'll read more about later in the book.

More than 80 autoimmune diseases have been identified, yet many are difficult to diagnose. Doctors generally treat symptoms, as a recognized cure for most autoimmune diseases has not yet been discovered.[2] I would like to note, however, that there are a number of biologic therapies for several of these diseases that work within the immune system to correct functionality. I would also like to note that at least some of these diseases can be addressed via diet and general wellness rather than modern biologics. Autoimmune diseases affecting children include:

- Type-1 diabetes
- Celiac disease
- Scleroderma
- Lupus
- Juvenile dermatomyositis
- Juvenile idiopathic rheumatoid arthritis
- AE/PANDAS (editor's note: Pediatric Autoimmune Neuropsychiatric Disease Associated with Strep Infection—PANDAS—is now generally diagnosed under the Autoimmune Encephalopathy umbrella)[3]

There are many others. These autoimmune diseases, in which the body starts reacting against, or attacking, itself, can

---

2 National Institutes of Health, U.S. Department of Health and Human Services Autoimmune Diseases (November 2012) www.niehs.nih.gov/health/materials/autoimmune_diseases_508.pdf (accessed April 2, 2019).

3 Carol Eustice, "Autoimmune Disease Types and Treatment," www.verywellhealth.com/what-is-an-autoimmune-disease-189661 (accessed April 22, 2019), and the American Autoimmune Related Diseases Association, Inc. www.aarda.org/diseaselist/ (accessed April 22, 2019).

Madeline R. Vann, MPH, "Childhood Autoimmune Disorders," www.everydayhealth.com/autoimmune-disorders/childhood-autoimmune-disorders.aspx (accessed April 22, 2019).

sometimes be difficult to recognize and assess. If you're not sure if your children have a predisposition to autoimmune disease, it's helpful to take a look at your family and ask, "Do we have allergies? Do we get Eczema? Do we get sick frequently? Do we have a history of anxiety or depression?"

Autoimmune diseases affect a large percentage of the population and tend to cluster among family members.

Autoimmune Disease and Mood Disorders

There is also a strong correlation between autoimmune diseases and anxiety, depression, ADHD, and ADD.[4] In a study published in 2018 by the *American Journal of Medical Genetics*, for instance, researchers observed significant genetic correlations between immune-related disorders and psychiatric disorders including anorexia nervosa, attention deficit-hyperactivity disorder, bipolar disorder, major depression, obsessive-compulsive disor-

---

4 William Cole, D.C., IFMCP, "The Issue That Could Be at the Root of Your Anxiety and Depression" www.mindbodygreen.com/0-21325/ the-issue-that-could-be-at-the-root-of-your-anxiety-depression. html (accessed April 22, 2019).

Yanjun Liu and Xiangqi Tang, "Depressive Syndromes in Autoimmune Disorders of the Nervous System: Prevalence, Etiology, and Influence," *Frontiers in Psychiatry* 9 (September 2018): 451. www. ncbi.nlm.nih.gov/pmc/articles/PMC6168717

Keith Loria, "Mental Health Condition Linked to Autoimmune Disease," *Managed Healthcare Executive* (November 2018) www. managedhealthcareexecutive.com/autoimmune-diseases/mental-health-condition-linked-autoimmune-disease (accessed April 22, 2019).

Jack Euesden et. al, "A bidirectional relationship between depression and the autoimmune disorders—New perspectives from the National Child Development Study," *PLoS One* 12, n. 3 (published online March 2017) www.ncbi.nlm.nih.gov/pmc/articles/PMC5338810/ (accessed April 22, 2019).

der, schizophrenia, smoking behavior, and Tourette syndrome.[5] Autoimmune disease may play a role in activating ADHD disorder. A study published in 2017 showed that autoimmune disease in the individual was associated with an increased risk of ADHD by an incidence rate ratio of 1.24 (95% CI 1.10-1.40). The researchers saw an association between maternal autoimmune disease and ADHD in a child.[6]

Researchers recently delved into Danish databases and found that 92,000 Danes born between 1945 and 1995 had been diagnosed with a mood disorder. Of these, 36,000—over one third—had suffered a severe infection or developed an autoimmune disease (such as Type 1 diabetes, celiac disease, lupus, and the like) at some point before being diagnosed with the mood disorder. According to the database, those who had been treated for a severe infection were 62% more likely to have developed a mood disorder than those who had never had one. An autoimmune disease increased the risk by 45%.[7]

Another scientific review published in the journal *Current Topics in Behavioral Neurosciences* in 2017 reported that up to 50%

5 Tylee, DS, "Genetic correlations among psychiatric and immune-related phenotypes based on genome-wide association data," *American Journal of Medical Genetics* 177, n. 7. (published online October 2018) https://onlinelibrary.wiley.com/doi/full/10.1002/ajmg.b.32652 (accessed June 25, 2019).

6 Nielsen, PR, "Associations Between Autoimmune Diseases and Attention-Deficit/Hyperactivity Disorder: A Nationwide Study," J Am Acad Child Adolesc Psychiatry. 2017 Mar;56(3):234-240. Published online 2016 Dec 27. https://www.ncbi.nlm.nih.gov/pubmed/28219489 (accessed June 25, 2019).

7 Skerrett PJ, "Infection, autoimmune disease linked to depression," *Harvard Health Blog* (June 2013) www.health.harvard.edu/blog/infection-autoimmune-disease-linked-to-depression-201306176397 (accessed May 6, 2019).

of patients with autoimmune diseases showed an impairment of health-related quality of life and exhibited depression-like symptoms. According to the researchers, the immune system leads to inflammation in affected organs and effects fatigue and depression-like symptoms via the body's timing system.[8]

Why Are These Diseases Becoming More Common?

The incidence of autoimmune disease has been increasing over the last several decades.[9] The National Institutes of Health (NIH) estimates that 23.5 million Americans are now affected. The American Autoimmune Related Diseases Association (AARDA) says it is much higher—more like 50 million.[10]

Why? Some experts say it's due to a changing environment. Our lifestyles are quite different today than they were a few decades ago. Most families, for example, are eating much more processed food than they did in the past. Children spend significantly less time outdoors. 85,000 chemicals are approved for use in commerce, and they aren't as well-tested as we believe.[11] Many of these chemicals may affect immune system function.

8 Pryce CR1, Fontana A, "Depression in Autoimmune Diseases." Curr Top Behav Neurosci. 2017;31:139-154. doi: 10.1007/7854_2016_7. https://www.ncbi.nlm.nih.gov/pubmed/27221625 (accessed June 3, 2019).

9 Schmidt CW, MS, "Questions Persist: Environmental Factors in Autoimmune Disease," *Environmental Health Perspectives* 119 n.6 (June 2011) www.ncbi.nlm.nih.gov/pmc/articles/PMC3114837/ (accessed April 2, 2019).

10 American Autoimmune Related Diseases Association, Inc. "Autoimmune Disease Statistics," www.aarda.org/news-information/statistics/ (accessed April 2, 2019).

11 Urbina I, "Think Those Chemicals Have Been Tested?" *The New York Times* (April 2013) www.nytimes.com/2013/04/14/sunday-review/think-those-chemicals-have-been-tested.html (accessed April 2, 2019).

While lifestyle changes such as vaccination, sanitation, and antibiotics have reduced instances of bacterial infections, there have also been unintended negative consequences that humans are just beginning to understand. All human beings are colonized by a number of bacteria equal to the number of their own cells. This creates an entire ecosystem inside of us, and we are beginning to unravel just how much we need these symbiotic bacteria to live healthfully.

Researchers and physicians are learning more each year about how gut health is associated with neurological disorders and autoimmune disease. For example, scientists at Queen's University found a specific gut microbe that makes molecules that influences the immune system to turn on its own cells.[12] The balance of gut bacteria is often different in patients with chronic inflammatory conditions (such as an autoimmune disorder) than in healthy individuals, [13] although it should be noted that a healthy gut microbiota varies considerably from person to person and changes in an individual over the course of their lifetime.

Intestinal bacteria help develop the immune system. Reduced exposure to these bacteria during infancy and childhood, therefore, may be influencing increased instances of immune and neurological disease later on in childhood.

The Sarkie Mazmanian lab hypothesizes that the human

---

12 "Researchers Discover New Link Between Autoimmune Diseases and a Gut Bacterium," *Infection Control Today* (October 2018) www.infectioncontroltoday.com/immune-system/researchers-discover-new-link-between-autoimmune-diseases-and-gut-bacterium (accessed May 6, 2019).

13 Kresser C, "Does the Gut Microbiome Play a Role in Autoimmune Disease?"
   chriskresser.com/does-the-gut-microbiome-play-a-role-in-autoimmune-disease (accessed May 6. 2019).

body depends on interactions with the products of our micro-biome. Researchers there are working to understand how the interaction between the beneficial gut microbiota and the immune and nervous systems may lead to natural therapeutics for human diseases.[14]

Since this is the cutting edge of scientific research, however, it may be years until these natural therapeutics become a mainstream part of Western medicine.

What Can We Do Now?

If you are struggling with an autoimmune or neurological disorder in your family such as AE, celiac, diabetes, or something related, you're probably not content to wait and hope for mainstream Western medicine to come up with an answer to these baffling conditions. Neither were we. Fortunately for our son, we encountered the right people at the right time to get him back to health.

This book explains how we did it—and how you can, too.

Today, you would not be able to detect the fierce battle our son fought and won. He is a healthy, athletic, scholarly and thriving child and we are so grateful for the return of his health and all that we have learned on our journey. It was an incredibly hard and emotional road. I feel it is my duty to get the word out about the tools and tactics that worked for us, and to share them with as many people as possible.

No one should have to go through this suffering. No child should have to go through such pain. No parent should be told to

---

14 "We All Live In A Microbial World," sarkis.caltech.edu (accessed April 2, 2019).

give up on their child and prepare to take care of their child for the rest of their lives. It is staggering to me how many "diseases" fall under an autoimmune umbrella, and how many of these have ties to mental health and the gut. So many terrifying health conditions and mental health struggles can be better addressed with diet and supplements—combined with typical Western medicine—than with conventional medicine alone.

That is the reason for this book. I hope you find it helpful.

1

OUR STORY

WHEN RYAN HAD A RUNNY and stuffy nose with a cough and mild fever during the second week of January, we kept him home from school for a few days. It was right after a wonderful and long holiday break, and everyone was slow to recover from the excitement. Nothing about our son's behavior struck us as unusual during that first week after he returned to school, but it is possible that we missed something. Teachers and coaches may have also been less tuned into his behavior than normal, after having been away from him over the holiday break.

About three weeks later, the last week of January, Ryan started constant uncontrollable eye-blinking that frustrated him and scared us. Then, a few days later, around February 1st, he had additional symptoms, tics that included incongruous shoulder shrugging, dull repeated throat clearing, and head turning.

Ryan began compulsively washing his hands, as much as 20-30 times per day. By about February 7th, he was displaying additional symptoms, including baby talk, loud nonsensical outbursts, continuously dilated eyes, thumb sucking, and clinginess. He even reverted to crawling—something he had not done for more than five years. Needless to say, this was not normal behavior for our child and we were quite alarmed.

From that point on, and for several months, Ryan complained of constant headaches, even though he had previously shown to have a very high pain tolerance.

Something's Not Right Here

My husband and I were scared. Ryan's teachers and everyone in our family had noticed something was seriously wrong with him. We took him to four different pediatricians in two weeks, hoping for help and answers. How could a normal, active, vivacious child turn into this? Over the course of four visits, we were told it was allergies, that "kids act funny sometimes," that it could possibly even be Tourette Syndrome. Finally, a fourth doctor said we needed to draw Ryan's blood for laboratory analysis.

Our son had been on antibiotics for two weeks in January to treat a sinus infection and possible Strep infection, but the doctors during those four visits never swabbed him. (I was also very sick the following week with what we believe to be the same thing.) Knowing what we know now, I can't help but wonder why screening for latent infection is not standard practice. As I wasn't feeling well myself, I was not equipped then to ask the right questions.

The Triggers: Bacterial and Viral Infections, Diet, and Genetic Predispositions

Years, research, and multiple doctors later, I now understand that it was a combination of genetics and environmental triggers that were making Ryan act so differently. According to the research, this is common. Your family might have an unknown genetic susceptibility to an autoimmune disorder that can influence neurological function, but nothing unusual may present itself until your child encounters triggers such as bacterial, viral, or fungal infections.

Multiple viruses have also been implicated in the diagnosis of autoimmune diseases. Those with a weakened immune system due to a poor diet are particularly vulnerable. According to *Autoimmunity: From Bench to Bedside* by María-Teresa Arango, Yehuda Shoenfeld, Ricard Cervera and Juan-Manuel Anaya, "Infections and exposure to pathogens or opportunistic organisms are among the environmental factors and may induce the initiation or exacerbation of autoimmune diseases. Many types of infection may influence one or more of these diseases, and a single organism may be able to trigger more than one autoimmune disease."[15]

There are multiple mechanisms by which host infection by a pathogen can lead to autoimmunity, according to a research review entitled "The role of infections in autoimmune disease" conducted by A. M. Ercolini and S. D. Miller and published in *Clinical & Experimental Immunology: The Journal of Translational Immunology* in 2009.

In the genetic makeup of many pathogens lie amino-acid sequences that mimic those in the cells of our own bodies. Under compromised conditions, the immune system cells that fight to combat these pathogens may confuse these same sequences as foreign, although they are normal components of our cells. Based

---

15 Arango, MT, et al., "Chapter 19: Infection and autoimmune diseases," *Autoimmunity: From Bench to Bedside* Bogota (Colombia): El Rosario University Press; 2013 Jul 18. www.ncbi.nlm.nih.gov/books/NBK459437/ (accessed April 22, 2019).

on molecular mimicry, such hyper-reactivity to self can result in an autoimmune cascade.[16]

What Else Has Been Shown to Trigger Autoimmune Responses?

Women represent an overwhelming 80% of autoimmune disorder patients; higher levels of hormones during the childbearing years could be a factor. Researchers at National Jewish Health have recently identified a specific trigger that helps explain why women suffer autoimmune disease more frequently. Age-associated B Cells (ABCs) have been found to drive autoimmune disease. The scientists conducting this study demonstrated that the transcription factor T-bet inside B cells causes ABCs to develop. When they deleted T-bet inside B cells, mice prone to develop autoimmune disease remained healthy. The researchers believe the same process occurs in humans with autoimmune disease, more often in elderly women.[17]

Scientists also believe injuries (for example, from regularly running long distances) may play a role in some types of autoimmune disease, as research has shown that an autoimmune response can happen after damage to tendons. As I mentioned previously, genetics play a role in autoimmune disease as well.

---

16 Ercolini AM & Miller SD, "The role of infections in autoimmune disease," *Clinical & Experimental Immunology* 155, n.1 (January 2009) 1-15. www.ncbi.nlm.nih.gov/pmc/articles/PMC2665673/ (accessed April 22, 2019).

17 National Jewish Health, "Trigger for autoimmune disease identified: Newly identified cells help explain why women suffer autoimmune disease more often." ScienceDaily, 10 May 2017. www.sciencedaily.com/releases/2017/05/170510174845.htm (accessed April 22, 2019).

Some families have multiple members affected by different autoimmune diseases.[18]

Our Story Continues

I look back and think about how this could've happened to Ryan. One of the clear and easily influenced aspects is diet and the absorption of the nutrients we are putting into our bodies—or failing to put in. Without a robust immune system, our families are more at risk for various illnesses than they should be. For instance, are we eating fruits and vegetables? Are we getting enough enzymes, complete omegas, enough vitamin B12, vitamin D3? Prebiotics? Probiotics? These are so integral to how our body functions.

By the end of February, the labs showed Ryan had higher than normal Strep titers (100-200 units/mL range). Titer means "concentration" or "unit." The labs also showed he had a Cytomegalovirus infection and Epstein-Barr Virus, as well as many vitamin/mineral levels well out of normal range (both extremely high and low).

Ryan's teacher was concerned enough that she asked a fellow parent who was a doctor to reach out to me and help our son. This parent was kind and explained the lab work. At the same time, the fourth pediatrician had given us a diagnosis and wanted to put our son on OCD/anti-tic medication. While we do believe in Western medicine, we were unwilling to accept the

18 "Autoimmune Disease: Why Is My Immune System Attacking Itself" reviewed by Ana-Maria Orbai, M.D., M.H.S. www.hopkinsmedicine.org/health/wellness-and-prevention/autoimmune-disease-why-is-my-immune-system-attacking-itself (accessed April 22, 2019).

fact that our son suddenly developed an obsessive-compulsive condition, neurological tics, developmental regression, and an utterly foreign personality literally overnight. There had to be a better explanation and a sensible and effective path to recovery. Psychiatric medication was not it. We weren't ready to put him on this type of medication without additional specialists, more information, and second or third opinions.

The Autoimmune-Neurological Connection

This was a very scary and lonely time for me and my family. Many people didn't understand what was happening to Ryan, and we barely had enough information to understand it ourselves, let alone explain it. Our friends and family were uncomfortable. We didn't know how to offer a rational explanation.

You might be wondering how we came to believe that Ryan had some sort of autoimmune disease rather than a strictly a neurological disorder, as we were being told. As I mentioned earlier, our questions among doctors and parents and research surfaced that they may be closely related, and conventional medicine is only just starting to look at the links. There was enough information to suggest there was more to find out and more we could do. The connection between our gut microbiome and the central nervous system (CNS) is a paradigm shift in neuroscience.[19] It may open new doors for ways to treat problems (including depression and anxiety) that have long been the purview of psychologists, not medical doctors.

---

19 Kelly JR, et al., "Breaking down the barriers: the gut microbiome, intestinal permeability and stress-related psychiatric disorders," *Frontiers in Cellular Neuroscience* 9 (October 2014). www.ncbi.nlm.nih.gov/pmc/articles/PMC4604320/ (accessed April 2, 2019).

Most important, to my mind, is the increasing recognition that mental health disorders are associated with low-grade systemic inflammation.[20] As we learn more about this connection, my hope is there will be new effective treatment protocols for many neurological disorders, including Alzheimer's and Parkinson's Disease.

Looking for Answers

Around that time, we used every last connection we had to get Ryan into the area Children's Hospital to see a neurologist. Unfortunately, the wait was about one month (down from normal three months), which seemed like an eternity.

Hour by hour and day by day, he got worse. By February 8th, we decided we weren't going to put up with waiting any longer. Ryan's tics were worse, his headaches were worse, and he was no longer recognizable as the boy we knew; in fact, he seemed to have no personality left at all. All we saw before us was a lost child with a blank stare who couldn't understand or communicate what was happening to him. He communicated dark thoughts of mortality—both his own and those close to him.

Even though I was unsure of how to explain my story, I was desperate, and so decided to reach out to a confidential support group for parents with children who had neurological conditions on Facebook, even though the idea of doing so scared me. Thankfully, the group's co-founder Kari spoke with me on the phone, and she was incredibly helpful (—her family's story is told in Chapter 4.)

---

20 Bested AC, et al., "Intestinal microbiota, probiotics and mental health: from Metchnikoff to modern advances: Part II—contemporary contextual research" *Gut Pathogens* 5 (published online March 2013). www.ncbi. nlm.nih.gov/pmc/articles/PMC3601973/ (accessed April 2, 2019).

Kari said, "You are not alone. You don't know me, but please put your son on antibiotics. Also, you have to get his tonsils out." She became a pivotal influence throughout our journey.

Kari gave me the name of a doctor who had treated hundreds of children with similar conditions all over the U.S. We sent this doctor Ryan's lab work, and he wanted more updated data. Within 24 hours of that phone call, Ryan was on cephalexin, a new antibiotic for him, along with olive leaf extract, a multivitamin, Omega-3s, and round-the-clock Motrin. Olive leaf extract contains bioactive compounds with antioxidant, antiatherogenic, anti-cancer, anti-inflammatory, and antimicrobial properties.[21]

We were ready to try anything.

A Turning Point

Within four days of that phone call (February 12th), and each and every day for the next five weeks, we saw a calmer child who was performing again at school. Ryan was still dealing with the constant eye blinking and headaches, however, and the light still hadn't returned to his eyes. His wild sense of humor wasn't back. He also grunted while trying to fall asleep and spent 12-14 hours per day sleeping. When he wasn't sleeping, he was tired and needed to rest on the couch. Given that Ryan's nickname had always been the Energizer Bunny, we knew we still had a long road ahead of us.

---

21 Omar, SH, "Cardioprotective and neuroprotective roles of oleuropein in olive" *Saudi Pharmaceutical Journal* 18, n. 3 (July 2010) 111-121. www.sciencedirect.com/science/article/pii/S131901641000040X (accessed April 2, 2019).

After about ten days, around mid-February, his new lab work ordered by the neurologist showed improved vitamin/mineral levels and decreasing Epstein-Barr and Cytomegalovirus levels. Unfortunately, the Strep titers were higher and now in the 200-300 units/mL range. So, Ryan was switched from cephalexin to Augmentin/azithromycin, and he improved more.

We were thrilled when we got in to see the specialist, Dr. Melanie Alarcio, a specialist in child neurology band pediatrics at Children's Hospital. I still remember thinking Ryan looked "too healthy" that day—my fear was the specialist would not believe there was a problem. I needn't have worried. He exhibited enough symptoms—twirling around, hand-washing, dilated eyes—that Dr. Alarcio could tell he was not in a normal state of neurologic health. She said they could cure him but it would be a long road. Dr. Alarcio drew eight vials of Ryan's blood, had us start a headache log, closely monitored Ryan's antibiotic regimen, asked us to schedule a tonsillectomy (even though he had healthy-looking tonsils); she also advised us to remove gluten and sugar from his diet.

Tonsils are two small masses of lymphoid tissue in the throat, on each side of the root of the tongue. Though the tonsils are part of the immune system, they can become chronically infected. In this case, they need to be removed.

Between these two doctors and the ENT specialist, we felt a degree of hope we hadn't felt in a long time. Ten days later, the lab work showed slow and steady increases in Ryan's health. One doctor explained we were going to "flip his immune system" and it would take a long time. Meanwhile, we were diligent and focused on learning everything we could about inflammation, infection, and genetics to ensure Ryan was on the path to normal levels.

The Long Road Back to Normal

It is amazing how seemingly difficult and monumental tasks and regimens at eventually became commonplace and routine for us. I remember thinking there was no way Ryan would take the antibiotics since they tasted terrible. Yet we got through that obstacle.

I remember him telling me, "Mommy, I can't swallow pills." He got over that as well.

I remember at first having to hold him down to draw his blood. Later, Ryan could have eight or nine vials of blood drawn at once without incident.

I remember thinking that all he wanted to eat was sugar and carbohydrates and him saying, "I'm not going to be gluten-free or have no sugar." We figured out a compromise and gave up gluten. Ryan now has sugar only once in a while.

The Tonsils Factor

In May, Ryan had his "healthy-looking" tonsils out. The tonsil microbiology showed a highly antibiotic-resistant form of a Strep. The Strep was resistant to clindamycin and Erythromycin. Once they were removed, we felt like we had gotten "the enemy." Dr. Alarcio switched Ryan to Ceftin on June 23rd. While he still had eye tics, by now they were minimal. The color in his cheeks came back and so did his sense of humor. His headaches were gone. We felt cautiously optimistic, but remained hyper-vigilant, and were even able to enjoy a family vacation together (medicine and all).

At this point, we were unsure of the best course of action, so we decided to stay the course. Research and literature showed the length of a given treatment really depended upon how long the child had been ill before they were treated. We had been prepared to plan for years, not months.

At the time, doctors were trying to figure out how to classify Ryan's illness, which was similar to Rheumatic Fever. Some say these cases can require years of antibiotics to ward off future infection and reduce inflammation. The doctors felt good about the fact that we had caught the problem within six weeks, but our son's immune system had a long way to go. We have truly learned how long it takes to rebuild one's immune system. Today, Ryan's illness would be classified as Autoimmune Encephalitis.

Chemical and Environmental Triggers

Inflammation became a large topic in our house and our lives. It was a major focus to seek out what causes inflammation and how to control and reduce it. This led us through a lot of research and discovery about environmental factors. Scientists are always learning more about autoimmune disease triggers, including environmental factors. For example, National Institute of Environmental Health Sciences (NIEHS) grantees recently took a look at what happens when mice are exposed to two autoimmune triggers at one time: trichloroethylene (a solvent and degreasing chemical) and mercuric chloride (a chemical used as a disinfectant). They found that disease development accelerated in the mice.[22]

_____

22 National Institutes of Health, U.S. Department of Health and Human Services Autoimmune Diseases (November 2012) www.niehs.nih.gov/health/materials/autoimmune_diseases_508.pdf (accessed April 2, 2019).

Gilbert, KM., "Coexposure to mercury increases immunotoxicity of trichloroethylene," _Toxicological Sciences_ 119 n. 2 (February 2011) www.ncbi.nlm.nih.gov/pubmed/21084432 (accessed April 2, 2019).

Other researchers studying the blood samples of mothers exposed to an environmental toxin passed on to humans by eating contaminated fish found elevated levels of antibodies in the blood of both the mothers and their fetuses.[23] In fact, one of the greatest risk factors for autoimmunity among women of childbearing age may be associated with exposure to mercury in the food supply, a recent University of Michigan study showed.[24]

I don't include this information to scare anyone—I just want readers to understand that the chemicals that are increasingly common in our environment have implications for the health of ourselves, our children, and increasing aging adult population. The world has changed in the past thirty years in ways that aren't always obvious...until you're dealing with a health crisis in your family and looking for the reasons why.

My Tonsillectomy

During the second half of the year that Ryan was sick, we heard reports of Strep "carriers" (meaning it is possible for a person to carry the infection and not be obviously ill) and had the entire families' labs pulled. Everyone was normal except for me. That was a serious blow. It turned out I had Strep titers in the 500-600 units/mL range, which is extremely high.

23 Nyland, JF et al., "Fetal and maternal immune responses to methylmercury exposure: a cross-sectional study" *Environmental Research* 111 n.4 (May 2011) www.ncbi.nlm.nih.gov/pubmed/21396635 (accessed April 2, 2019).

24 Somers, E, et al., "Mercury Exposure and Antinuclear Antibodies among Females of Reproductive Age in the United States: NHANES." *Environmental Health Perspectives*, 2015; DOI: www.sciencedaily.com/releases/2015/02/150210050438.htm (Accessed April 2, 2019).

I went on and off antibiotics from June to February and strangely felt better in terms of energy, mood, and ability to multitask while on the antibiotics. This was my own personal experience seeing how our physical health (and low-grade illness and inflammation) impacts our mental health.

Unfortunately, during this time I repeatedly had my labs pulled and the titer never moved. The antibiotics weren't really touching the problem. Thus, I made the difficult decision to undergo an expensive, painful surgery to have my tonsils removed. Additionally, given my history of sinus infections, I decided to simultaneously undergo nasal surgery as well. I had suffered repeatedly since the age of 12 with sinus infections and Strep throat a few times a year. As a result, taking this step didn't seem that far-fetched to me.

The pathology report of my tonsils showed acute tonsillitis with lots of bacteria and debris. Unfortunately, they "forgot" to culture the tonsils despite being repeatedly asked. Four weeks after the tonsillectomy, my lab work showed my strep markers (ASO and Anti-DNase B) ASO went from 224 to 184 to 170 and Anti-DNase B went from 560 to 312 to 348. I redo labs every 12 months to monitor. What I think is an interesting by-product of this procedure is I haven't had a sinus infection since the surgery and I don't crave sugar the way I once did.

How Essential Oils Help Our Family

The next year around the holidays, Ryan was a lot better. However, he still wouldn't have playdates with kids if he noticed didn't wash their hands after they used the restroom, and he was scared of anyone who was sick or didn't feel well. As time went on, each year later, we noticed certain things would set off his symptoms again, which always scared us, and still does. For instance, we tended to notice tics and loud behavior about 24–48 hours before a note came home from school that Strep was found in his grade level. (We were very fortunate that the school worked with us and shared any contagious illnesses when they happened.)

In the two to three years following diagnosis, we were usually able to get by with Motrin to reduce the sudden tics every six hours for three to seven days, but every once in a while, there was a strep infection in the school that particularly bothered Ryan and a 10-day course of Cefdinir (a cephalosporin antibiotic) would set him back on course. Azithromycin (a macrolide-type antibiotic) had no effect on him.

Two years after his original successful treatment, we found that by introducing essential oils supplementation (particularly frankincense, oregano, cinnamon, turmeric, clove, and copaiba), Ryan did NOT experience these triggers the same way. His immune system could fight the infections that would make others around him sick. We also became diligent about taking a daily probiotic, B12, methylfolate, and vitamin D3 to make the immune system stronger and balance his mood.

Fast forward several years later: we are happy that we don't have setbacks anymore.

While some people hear "essential oils" and roll their eyes, I'd encourage you to keep an open mind on the topic. Frankincense, for example, has been used in traditional and modern natural medicine for the treatment of a variety of illnesses with very minimal side effects. A recent scientific review of this resin published in the *Journal of Traditional and Complementary Medicine* showed its anti-inflammatory, anti-arthritic, anti-proliferative, antimicrobial, and analgesic effects. Frankincense reduces inflammation and pain in the body and relieves the related symptoms of many diseases.[25]

Science is also showing how beneficial essential oils can be when they are used in concert with probiotics. According to a review article entitled, "Development of Probiotic Candidate in Combination with Essential Oils from Medicinal Plant and Their Effect on Enteric Pathogens: A Review" conducted at the School of Biochemical Engineering at the Indian Institute of Technology, probiotics and essential oils both have a great potential in terms of their beneficial effect against microbial gut infection. They also show a synergistic effect that is higher than any known drug due to their complementary actions.[26]

Plant extracts are going mainstream. A recent piece in *The Atlantic* entitled "Essential Oils Might Be the New Antibiotics" explains why. Because bacteria are increasingly drug-resistant, scientists and farmers are now looking to plant extracts (essential oils) to control infection.[27] It's easy to hear the phrase "drug-resistant bacteria" and shrug it off as media

25 Hamidpour R, et. al., "Frankincense: From the Selection of Traditional Applications to the Novel Phytotherapy for the Prevention and Treatment of Serious Diseases," *Journal of Traditional and Complementary Medicine* 3, n. 4 (October-December 2013) www.ncbi. nlm.nih.gov/pmc/articles/PMC3924999/ (accessed April 2, 2019).

26 Shipradeep S, et al. "Development of Probiotic Candidate in Combination with Essential Oils from Medicinal Plant and Their Effect on Enteric Pathogens: A Review" *Gastroenterology Research and Practice* 2012. www.hindawi.com/journals/grp/2012/457150/ (accessed April 2, 2019).

27 Tori Rodriguez, "Essential Oils Might be the New Antibiotics," *The Atlantic* (January 2015) www.theatlantic.com/health/archive/2015/01/the-new-antibiotics-might-be-essential-oils/384247 (accessed May 6, 2019).

fear-mongering, but to people who really understand the issue, the problem is a clear and present danger.[28] In response to it, the food industry and healthcare practitioners are looking at essential oils. Because they have antimicrobial, antibacterial, and antifungal properties, these extracts are being used in the food industry as natural preservatives.[29] They can also be used instead of antibiotics to keep animals in our food supply healthy. For example, a study published in 2014 found that chickens who were given feed with added oregano oil had a 59% lower mortality rate due to a common infection in poultry than untreated chickens.[30]

You'll read more on this topic in Chapter 8 of this book. I've become so convinced of the efficacy of essential oils and other key supplements to bolster our immune system that I've worked with doctors to develop two new products for families called Hello Health.

The two supplements we've created combine the best probiotics, vitamins, and essential oils to keep kids' and adults' immune systems, brain and mood functioning optimally.

---

28 "Antimicrobial Resistance: Tackling a crisis for the health and wealth of nations," *The Review on Antimicrobial Resistance* Chaired by Jim O'Neill (December 2014) amr-review.org/ (accessed May 6, 2019).

29 Bomgardner MM, "Extending Shelf Life with Natural Preservative," *Chemical & Engineering News* 92, n. 6 (February 2014). cen.acs.org/articles/92/i6/Extending-Shelf-Life-Natural-Preservatives.html (accessed May 6, 2019).

30 Betancourt L, et al., "Effect of Origanum chemotypes on broiler intestinal bacteria," *Poultry Science* 93, n. 10 (October 2014) 2526-2535. academic.oup.com/ps/article/93/10/2526/1535580 (accessed May 6, 2019).

The Right Medical Team

We were very fortunate to have found a psychologist famil-
iar with long-term childhood illnesses who helped our family
talk through the ups, downs, and struggles of what we were going through. We had no idea how lonely that road would feel.
Our psychologist has been paramount to our family's recovery.
However, I do want to caution any reader whose child's behavior has abruptly changed. Yes, please do consult a psychologist
or psychiatrist. But be sure to look at root physiological causes
as well. You need to have the whole picture before (or instead
of) turning to psychoactive drugs. I say this because while we
were so fortunate to have a good team of doctors around us—Dr.
Trifiletti, Dr. Alarcio, Dr. Casper, and Dr. Peterson—it is sad
that for three years we were called on the phone by our former pediatrician and former neurologist and told that Ryan had
Tourette Syndrome, and that he should be taken off antibiotics
and Motrin and put on mind-altering medication.

What these doctors failed to understand is Ryan didn't have
any symptoms when he was on Motrin and/or antibiotics. If he
truly had Tourette Syndrome, the antibiotics and Motrin would
have had no effect on his behavior. I must admit, however, if I
hadn't seen this myself, I may never have believed it either.

A New Conversation about Neurological Health

We recently heard on the news that Child Protective Services
had been called on a mother by someone who didn't believe in
her preferred course of treatment. It's time to change the conversation on this heartbreaking state of affairs.

There is a large community of parents who are going through what we went through and are scared to address and talk about it for fear of backlash from the medical community. For anyone who says an illness can't cause neurological issues, just ask a mother who feeds her child corn syrup or red dye if her child acts differently afterward. I ask that we all take a step back and recognize the mind-body connection and communicate what is right for pediatric health. We need to understand the system interactions and *why* an illness may cause neurological issues rather than debate *if* an illness could cause neurological issues.

We continue to be so thankful that we were among the lucky few that came out the other side of this health crisis. We have learned about genetic mutations, how to avoid triggers, and protect our son's body through the use of better nutrients—both in the form of food and with supplements and essential oils. We have learned about gut health and the blood-brain barrier, autoimmune disorders, and how it may all tie together—or fall apart—when bacterial, viral or fungal infections present themselves.

Additionally, I am encouraged and closely watching the new research coming out regarding infections and their tie with Alzheimer's disease.[31] Researchers are looking at whether certain viruses, bacteria, or fungal infections can cause or are correlated to Alzheimer's disease. Some research shows Alzheimer's is more common in people who have these infections; for example, evidence of herpes infection has been found in the parts of the

---

31 Bibi, F., "Link between chronic bacterial inflammation and Alzheimer disease," *CNS & Neurological Disease Drug Targets* 13, n. 7 (2014) www.ncbi.nlm.nih.gov/pubmed/25230225 (accessed April 22, 2019).

brain that are particularly affected in Alzheimer's disease. In addition, the bacteria that causes pneumonia has been found inside the brain cells of people with Alzheimer's disease.[32]

There is also some new evidence that the condition is caused by a bacterium involved in gum disease. A bacterial hypothesis for Alzheimer's doesn't mean your genetic makeup doesn't matter as well. The human body's genetic predisposition for inflammation varies from person to person. Chronic inflammation can affect our immune systems, and this may influence how much damage *P. gingivalis* induces. This fresh finding could help scientists create effective treatments or even a vaccine.[33]

If you're going through a health scare involving behavioral or mental health changes with your own child, I have many helpful hints. First, let's look at some of the latest research on this topic and the problem with the healthcare status quo.

---

32 "Could treating infections prevent or treat Alzheimer's?" Alzheimer's Society: United Against Dementia www.alzheimers.org.uk/about-dementia/risk-factors-and-prevention/infections-and-dementia (accessed April 22, 2019).

33 MacKenzie, D, "We may finally know what causes Alzheimer's—and how to stop it," *New Scientist* (January 2019) www.newscientist.com/article/2191814-we-may-finally-know-what-causes-alzheimers-and-how-to-stop-it/ (accessed April 22, 2019).

2

THE FOUNDATION OF GOOD HEALTH

SCIENTIFIC RESEARCH REVEALS A STRONG link between what we consume and how we feel mentally and emotionally.[34] For example, vitamin B12-related markers are associated with total brain volume, according to a cross-sectional review of research published in the journal *Neurology*.[35]

It might be time to think of supplements, fruits, vegetables, and plant extracts as medicines.

A study of more than 12,000 Australians conducted between 2007 and 2013, published in the *American Journal of Public Health* in 2016, found that people who increased the number of servings of fruits and vegetables that they ate reported they were happier and more satisfied with their life than those whose

34 Schiffman, R., "Can What We Eat Affect How We Feel?" *The New York Times,* March 2019. www.nytimes.com/2019/03/28/well/eat/food-mood-depression-anxiety-nutrition-psychiatry.html (accessed April 8, 2019).

35 Tangney, C.C., "Vitamin B12, cognition, and brain MRI measures: A cross-sectional examination," *Neurology* 77, n. 13 (September 2011). n.neurology.org/content/77/13/1276 Accessed April 8, 2019.

diets remained the same. The impact was similar to moving from unemployed to employed.[36] I once had a health and wellness expert tell me, "Live food makes you feel better than dead food." However, I admit I find it hard to get enough fruits and vegetables in my and my family's diet so we do rely a lot on smoothies.

Research is also showing the critical role of omega-3 fatty acids in the function of the central nervous system and in the outcomes of depression. According to a paper entitled "Omega-3 fatty acids and major depression: A primer for the mental health professional," the dietary intake of Omega-3 fatty acids has decreased substantially in Western countries over the last century. The Standard American Diet currently has omega-6 fats outnumbering omega-3s by a ratio of up to 20:1, yet the ideal dietary ratio of Omega-6 to Omega-3 has been recommended by an international panel of lipid experts to be approximately 2:1. Omega-3 fatty acids are found in seafood and several nut and seed oils. Epidemiological studies support a connection between dietary fish/seafood consumption and a lower prevalence of depression.[37]

Given this information, I don't want to just focus on Autoimmune Encephalopathy in this book. I want to start raising questions around a number of diseases: "Hey, here's some research about mental health and diet, here's some new

36 Redzo Mujcic, Ph.D. & Andrew J. Oswald, DPhil, "Evolution of Well-Being and Happiness After Increases in Consumption of Fruit and Vegetables," *AJPH Research* 106, n.8 (August 2016) warwick.ac.uk/fac/soc/economics/intranet/manage/news/ajph_actual_july_2016_fruit_and_veg_oswald_final_proofs.pdf (accessed April 8, 2019).

37 Logan, AC, "Omega-3 fatty acids and major depression: A primer for the mental health professional," *Lipids in Health and Disease* 3 (November 2004). www.ncbi.nlm.nih.gov/pmc/articles/PMC533861/ (accessed April 8, 2019).

data on irritable bowel syndrome, here's some research about Alzheimer's." I want all of us to consider and be open to hearing about how all of these conditions overlap, and the things we can do in our own homes with diet and supplements to stay healthy—and to keep our children's minds and bodies healthy.

Depression is the top cause of disability in Americans between the ages of 15 and 44, according to the World Health Organization.[38] It affects nearly 10% of the adult population in the U.S., and only one in ten adults eat federal recommendations for daily fruit and vegetable consumption. The interesting thing is that these recommended amounts aren't even that high—just 1 ½ to 3 cups per day, depending on age. According to the Centers for Disease Control, high cost, limited availability and access, and perceived lack of cooking/preparation time can be barriers to fruit and vegetable consumption in the U.S. [39]

I recognize these barriers, but nevertheless, the science is becoming louder and clearer. A recent study with over 400 participants in New Zealand and the United States, for example, found that providing young adults aged 18-25 with high-quality fresh fruits and vegetables resulted in significant short-term improvements to their psychological well-being.[40]

---

38 "Mood Disorders," National Institutes of Health Fact Sheet report. nih.gov/NIHfactsheets/ViewFactSheet.aspx?csid=48&key=M (accessed April 8, 2019).

39 "Only 1 in 10 Adults Get Enough Fruits or Vegetables," Centers for Disease Control and Prevention www.cdc.gov/media/releases/2017/p1116-fruit-vegetable-consumption.html (accessed April 8, 2019).

40 Conner, TS, "Let them eat fruit! The effect of fruit and vegetable consumption on psychological well-being in young adults: A randomized controlled trial," *PLOS ONE* (February 2017) journals.plos.org/plosone/article?id=10.1371/journal.pone.0171206 (accessed April 8, 2019).

What is the Main Story the Research is Trying to Tell Us?

Scientists and researchers are just beginning to understand the complex interplay between our food choices, our gut microflora, our genetics, our immune functions, and our brain health. For example, serotonin is a key neurotransmitter. The gut microbiome is critical to the normal functioning of the gut-brain axis, and behavior linked to serotonergic neurotransmission has been shown to be influenced by gut microbiota. The gut microbiota is, therefore, an emerging therapeutic target.[41]

Could it be that when our bodies are nutritionally starved, we're more susceptible to triggers, bacterial and viral, that bring on these genetic expressions to disease? Perhaps this is why we see this major uptick in autism and autoimmune problems—and not only these, but in anxiety and depression as well.

Now, I'd like to introduce another family with a similar story to ours.

Deborah's Journey and Success Story

First and foremost, I would like to thank Pamela for giving me the opportunity to share my son's story. During the summer of 2005, we almost lost him to what is now being referred to as Autoimmune Encephalopathy. I am also grateful that Pamela has decided to write this book and share the knowledge she has

---

41 O'Mahony, SM, et al., "Serotonin, tryptophan metabolism and the brain-gut-microbiome axis," *Behavioural Brain Research* 277, n. 15 (January 2015): 32-48. www.sciencedirect.com/science/article/pii/S0166432814004768 (accessed April 8, 2019).

gained connecting physical wellbeing and mental disorders. My heartfelt gratitude also goes to Dr. Susan Swedo, the Chief of the Pediatrics and Developmental Neuroscience Branch at the US National Institute of Mental Health, for her dedicated perseverance research on PANDAS. Dr. Swedo is currently the Chief of the PANDAS Physician Network (PNN) after retiring from the NIMH in April 2019, as Scientist Emeritus.

As for me, I am a degreed biologist, allied health scientist, and have worked in consumer product research and regulatory affairs for 25 years prior to teaching science at a top, very rigorous STEM charter school. I am considered a "Subject Expert Teacher" and teach basic biology, chemistry, physics, and AP Environmental Science. I have been teaching for the last 14 years. I see so many Strep infections, so many children (in the 5TH grade level) with blank looks, pale complexions, unable to do simple math, unable to write on a line or even draw a picture. Several students have come in and actually pulled up their shirts to show me their rash and tell me the doctor said they have scarlet fever. These children are diagnosed with OCD, Tourette's, ADHD, ADD, learning disabilities, everything but PANDAS or PANS. They take several different kinds of mind-altering medicines but not one is on an antibiotic long term. As a biologist and mother of a child that had PANDAS, I know what it looks like.

My son is now 24 years old and was "cured" of PANDAS in 2005 when Dr. Susan Swedo, of the National Institute of Mental Health, suggested a full year of antibiotics. If it were not for the quick "diagnosis" and treatment he would not be the intelligent, courageous, young man he is today. We saw over 10 doctors in a 6-week period that summer of 2005. One doctor finally listened and learned. I took in Dr. Swedo's research papers and shared her hypothesis on PANDAS. This doctor actually called Dr. Swedo and prescribed the antibiotic for a year that saved my son. The prescription was written for laryngitis, not PANDAS.

The medical profession is treating the symptoms not the cause.

My son had several Strep throat infections and sinus infections every year between about six to 10 years of age. One day, he woke up with a slight sore throat and little, if any, fever. I called his doctor and they said a virus was going around—and NOT to bring him in. He stayed home from school that day and I remember him having a weird nightmare. It was not until about six weeks later that his "episodes" began.

The first thing that happened was screaming. I grabbed him, held him, and sang to him, tried to calm him, but nothing worked until we left the room. He would not talk about why he was so upset—he simply trembled with fear. I made his favorite dinner that evening, spaghetti with red sauce, yet he could not eat it. The spaghetti fell out of his mouth. He told me it was blood and that he could not eat it.

My heart pounded. What was happening to my strong, outgoing little spaghetti-eater? I suggested we go outside for a walk, but he could not go farther than the porch. He was physically unable to move past the cracks in the sidewalk. He trembled. He was white, pale, colorless. His pupils were huge.

He kept turning his bedroom light on and off and he repeatedly opened and closed doors in our home. He needed to be by my side. Separation was not an option—I had to lay next to him in his bed and hold his hand even though he was ten years old. It was days later that he could finally tell me of "Bloody Mary" in the mirror. He told me that if he (my son) did not kill his mother (me), "Bloody Mary" was going to kill him. I can still remember the voice "kill mother"—it came from my son, but it was not HIM.

What was happening to my son? I stayed up most of the next several nights, searching for answers. I learned about OCD— Obsessive Compulsive Disorder—and read one line about a possible connection between Strep infections and OCD behavior. I learned about PANDAS, which stands for Pediatric Autoimmune Neuropsychiatric Disorders Associated with Streptococcal Infections [editor's note: PANDAS is now under the umbrella of an Autoimmune Encephalopathy diagnosis], thanks to the National Institute of Mental Health and Dr. Susan Swedo's research. Her work was still in its infancy at that time.

I called my son's pediatrician and made an appointment. I talked with hospitals and with specialists who told me to bring him down to the hospital. They said he needed to be "evaluated," but my mother's intuition said no. I told them I want a blood test—the one that could tell me if his Strep titer is high. The doctors said he could not possibly have anything like PANDAS.

The doctors were in denial. Fortunately, after I *insisted* that a blood test be taken, they agreed. A couple days later, I got a call. His blood titer was high—very high. The PA, physician assistant, said, "Can you bring him down…now? Let's give him a shot of penicillin."

They put him on some antibiotics and he was better within days. When the antibiotics were gone, his symptoms returned. I took him to several psychiatrists. They prescribed Abilify and Prozac, mind altering drugs. They did not help.

I told the doctors, "the specialists" that he needed antibiotics, but they said, "No, we can't keep him on antibiotics long term." Apparently, however, they *could* keep him on mind altering drugs long term. Why? They were not helping. They wanted to "try" different kinds of psychiatric drugs. I felt strongly that this approach was wrong. My feeling was, "No! The Strep it is still there—somewhere. Find it and get rid of it."

They asked if he still had his tonsils and said he should have them taken them out. At that time, the NIMH said they did not think there was a connection. I was thinking, "Don't tonsils help fight germs?"

When he got Strep, the infection appeared to be in the back of his throat and his sinuses, not in his tonsils. We took him to two ENT specialists who said his tonsils were healthy and they would not remove them.

My son would tell me of the voice, of how he knew he should stop opening and closing doors, and stop turning lights on and off, but he couldn't stop. He told me he was afraid of what the voice was telling him to do. "Mommy, mommy!" he would cry, scream out in fear. "PLEASE make it stop. Mommy help me... make it go away." There was so much fear and pain in his voice.

In just a few days, I was losing him. He was white, pale, colorless. He had fear in his beautiful blue eyes. No emotion was left except fear, OCD, and tic-like movements. I discovered later that St. Vitus's dance, called Sydenham's chorea (a childhood neurological disorder), has been linked to Strep. My son had similar movements at times.

I felt desperate. *How do we get him back?* Finally, one doctor called NIMH, after I had given him Dr. Swedo's research papers. He prescribed an antibiotic for laryngitis, for an entire year, as was suggested by Dr. Swedo. This saved my son. No more psychiatrists, no more mind-altering drugs, just straight old penicillin. His color came back and he returned to himself in days. However, his brain did need time to heal. My son was back. His eyes were open with hope not fear, with a strong desire to live and love again. His mind was healing. On penicillin, there were no more tears, no outbursts, no debilitating OCD, no tics, no more opening and closing of doors.

My son was "cured" of his illness in 2005 after a full year of antibiotics. I also give him Motrin if he became "moody" and daily supplements such as omega-3 and a multi-vitamin. He periodically took sinus/allergy over-the-counter medication. As a teen, he had acne and was prescribed antibiotics. It is my opinion that this combination helped keep the inflammation in his brain under control.

My suggestion to anyone reading this book is to *never* give up hope. Never give up on finding the correct diagnosis and treatments for your child. You know your child better than anyone else. Keep records of changes in behavior, temperament, anxiety, appetite, writing and math skills. But *never* give up! I have been fortunate to be able to share my story through education and as an advocate for PANDAS. Many parents listen and have been able to "save" their child. It can be a battle, but with books like this, along with medical research and further education, we can make the shift that is so desperately needed. The quick, correct diagnosis and treatments are essential to obtain a healthy mind and body for all children.

My son graduated with honors from university in Genetics, Cell and Developmental Biology and volunteered at a biomedical facility in 2017. His research focused on genetics and environmental factors which may cause schizophrenia. He is currently finishing up his second year working towards his PhD in neuroscience in the College of Molecular Biology and Biomedical Sciences at a top medical school. His current research focuses on pediatric mental disorders and genetics. Below are a few words taken from his college acceptance letter back in 2013:

> *My intellectual endeavor is to study the neural aspect of the brain for a signal that could help determine why some children obtain OCD symptoms after Strep throat infections. Research has shown that these illnesses and mental disorders are somehow connected; however, the entire connection needs to be discovered. I want to find the causes that link these seemingly harmless sicknesses to their extreme and detrimental mental disorders. By studying the brain, behaviors, and the correlation with bacterial infections, I hope to discover the cure or at least, a warning signal. I envision the ability to read symptoms and signs of an oncoming episode that can be deterred and ultimately stopped. Finding these signals may lead to finding cures for various types of mental disorders.*
>
> *A seemingly hopeless period of time in the summer of 2005 is now what inspires me to provide hope for others. With my future work in the field of neuroscience, I will take my past experiences to create a better future for others.*

We were fortunate to have found a pediatrician who finally listened. We are grateful that Dr. Swedo emailed a response (I still have her email) and that the doctor prescribed the antibiotic. My son still takes a daily multi-vitamin and probiotic and eats a very health-conscious diet. We support keeping the brain and body healthy with the help of diet, supplements, and an educated medical community. Please, never give up.

3

Changing
the Healthcare
Status Quo

From a higher level, people in healthcare are not being exposed to multiple ways of healing. Based on my experiences, I feel comfortable saying that doctors are not 100% well-informed when it comes to the latest research on autoimmune triggers and the link between our gut and our mental health. For example, the head of the pediatric doctor's group that I encountered said there was no way that viruses and bacteria could break through the blood-brain barrier. This was years ago. In that time, thankfully, there's been research and that information has been debunked. You'll read more about the blood-brain barrier in Dr. Alarcio's chapter.

Doctors have been educated to believe, in many cases, that the mind and the body are separate. It's very important to realize, and for doctors to be educated, that there is a connection between what happens in our physical body and what happens mentally.

Healthcare Customization and Genetic Testing

There is a lot of talk now about treating each patient as unique and customizing a healing plan for the person, not "one size fits all." This is becoming more realistic with the accessibility of affordable genetic testing at local pharmacies and companies like 23andme. The ability to take the raw data to doctors that understand how to interpret and treat the person, as well as using sites such as geneticgenie.org, help make this possible.

We ran 23andme raw data into geneticgenie.org and found it matched 100% to the expensive blood results our family members had undergone. With additional education and training, perhaps every person can be better informed about themselves and ask the right questions when we are choosing and receiving healthcare. We really need to be looking at each person's genetic history for a customized treatment plan. It's actually becoming cost-effective.

Integrative and Functional Medicine

There are also more doctors who look at the whole person instead of just a list of symptoms. These are called integrative or functional doctors. An integrative physician, according to Beth Lambert's book *Brain Under Attack*, is one who takes all aspects of a person into account when developing a treatment plan— mind, body, and spirit. An integrative doctor will use Western, or conventional, healing modalities and medicines as well as alternative approaches.

Similarly, functional medicine looks at a whole person and their comprehensive health history. A functional medicine practitioner looks for root causes of chronic health problems and works with patients to address these causes (there are usually several). Functional medicine doctors regularly recommend dietary and lifestyle changes in addition to traditional treatments.

Climbing Over the Wall of Confusion

Our son was not acting normally when he got so sick. It was very scary, and the first doctors we saw about it were not helpful. Again, he was baby talking, crawling, devoid of all emotion.

We kept going back to the doctors (nearly half a dozen times in two weeks), and they kept saying things like, "Oh, kids will be kids," or "Don't worry about it, this is a phase. It'll pass," or "It could be a viral infection, it'll run its way out." One doctor said, "That looks kind of serious. Why don't we send him to a psychologist and have them take a look?" Another said, "Can you call and get an appointment at the local Children's Hospital?" (Which takes three to six months.)

They just didn't know what to do. And it's not their fault. They haven't been comprehensively educated in some of these autoimmune symptoms, genetic mutations, and the overlap between our physiology and mental health.

The MTHFR Mutation

I hear more and more from parents whose kids are experiencing anxiety and depression. There's a genetic enzyme mutation they can actually test for now that allows you to find out if you have a predisposition to anxiety, depression, heart disease, autoimmune disorders. It is very common, affecting up to 40% of the population.

MTHFR is the acronym for an enzyme (methylenetetrahydrofolate reductase) that may play a key role in many aspects of emotional and physical health. If you have this particular mutation, you may be predisposed to the most common mental conditions as well as other health problems including migraines, strokes and cardiovascular disease. This mutation may prevent you from properly absorbing vitamins and minerals and shedding toxins. It can also alter your response to some medications.

One reason this enzyme is so important is it converts folate into a useable form for your body.[42] When this process is disrupted, our neurotransmitters are affected. Therefore, if you do have this mutation, you can take action. For example, instead of taking a supplement with folic acid, you can take one with a more bioavailable form called l-methylfolate. You can also eat a diet rich in folate.[43] You can enjoy more greens like spinach, okra, and turnip greens. For the highest levels of bio-available B vitamins, turn to organ meats like chicken liver or grass-fed beef liver.

A lot of this is tied together, to the point that I believe, over the next couple of decades, we're going to start to understand so much more about how you treat your body and how that affects your mind. What you eat, what nutrients you receive, plays

---

42 William Cole, D.C. IFMCP, "What You Need to Know about the Gene Mutation that Affects 40% of the Word," www.mindbodygreen. com/0-21657/what-you-need-to-know-about-the-gene-mutation-that-affects-40-of-the-world.html (accessed May 6, 2019).

43 Traci Stein Ph.D., MPH, "A Genetic Mutation That Can Affect Mental & Physical Health: MTHFR mutations are linked to depression, ADHD, migraines, miscarriage & more," *Psychology Today* (September 2014). www.psychologytoday.com/us/blog/the-integrationist/201409/genetic-mutation-can-affect-mental-physical-health (Accessed May 6, 2019).

a large role in determining how your body will cope with and shed the high levels of toxicity that we come into contact with on a daily basis, as well as the bacterial and the viral infections we come into contact with. Our bodies, with fully functioning immune systems, can combat these things and not allow them to run rampant through your body, affecting how you feel and how you think.

As genetic testing improves, we'll need to keep asking: what other mutations are common that are correlated with autoimmune and neurological and nervous disorders?

Is Healthcare Serving Patients?

This is something we need additional research on, but I am concerned about the medical schools in the United States being heavily influenced by the pharmaceutical companies. In talking to the people I know who live in Europe, especially in Germany, whenever they get an infection and the doctor gives them an antibiotic, they are also given a probiotic, a B12 and a D3 supplement to take along with it. Because that antibiotic is getting rid of both bad and good stuff, you need to make sure that your body has what it needs to heal.

Here in the United States, I just don't think most pediatricians have 100% of the information. When they come out of school, they figure "I got this!" But there's so much more to it.

Meeting Dr. Alarcio

Dr. Melanie Alarcio, a pediatric neurologist who uses an integrative whole-person approach to treating her patients, helped heal my son. I still remember being so frightened in her office the very first time. My son was twirling around, around, and around. His eyes were dilated. He couldn't stop. He kept humming and had to go wash his hands a few times. My husband and I, we were scared to death. The other doctor had told us to prepare ourselves to take care of him for the rest of our lives.

I pulled a personal favor and got him in with her. And she said, "Don't worry, I'm going to cure him." Tears came to my eyes. I was like, "Oh my God, thank you so much. I don't know how, I am so scared right now, but thank you."

It was such a breakthrough for us. Dr. Alarcio is a trained neurologist who knows traditional medicine and can exercise traditional medicine but is open to alternatives as well. She treats each patient as an individual. She goes deep and asks questions like, "Can we pull blood tests and look at what's going on?" One size does not fit all.

She looks at supplements and diet. There's more and more talk in the circles I'm starting to associate with of parents who are looking for integrative medicine. What is traditional? What is functional? What is integrative? I think a lot of us have questions about this as we're going out and finding doctors. What does that mean? Who should I be going to? Are they going to look at me as a person? Are they trained to give me what I need? Those questions are really scary when you have something serious going on with your child.

What is really upsetting to me is I have a close friend who told me a few weeks ago that her son was having tics. And it's like, okay that happens. It could be that he's had a trigger, he could be reacting to something. Then she told me a few days ago that he wanted to commit suicide. I was like, "Look, I've been there, done that. He is having a severe reaction and you need to get his body under control, and here are some things I think you should do. I think you should restrict his diet and take away some of the stuff that could be feeding the problem, like the sugar."

I think I managed to send her in a different direction, which is fortunate, but I hear stories like this all the time that concern me. She made an appointment with a psychologist, and I said, "Listen, a psychologist is only one piece of what you need right now." It is important for family healing once you've got a hand around how to help this child, but it really breaks my heart that people are missing so much of what could be the root cause of the problem in the meantime.

Antibiotics

The antibiotics they initially had my son on were the wrong ones. This is the hard part when it comes to understanding how best to treat a child. Unless they test the bacteria in the infection, they have no idea what the right antibiotic is. When they pulled out my son's tonsils and cultured them, they found a type of bacteria that was highly resistant and could not be touched by standard antibiotics like amoxicillin. So, all of that dosing was for naught. At one point his kidneys were showing "distress" at long-term antibiotic and Advil use. It would be really nice if they could find an easy way to test the bacteria and get back to you instead of just handing you a Z-pack. The short answer, for now, is there is no easy way to do this.

IVIG

Intravenous immunoglobulin is a standard treatment for individuals with autoimmune disorders (antibody deficiencies), and it was one I wanted to avoid for my son if at all possible. How it works is they take healthy cells from up to 10,000 or 15,000 donors and pump them into your body.[44] The healthy cells kill your cells, basically helping the body reboot. But this treatment doesn't last forever and it's incredibly expensive.

I thought, why would I put a port into a child, which would be incredibly traumatic for him, as well as opening up another potential bacteria source, which seems dangerous, and it's not permanent? Yet this is the normal protocol. I was like, *there's got to be a better way.*

---

44 Jolles. S., et al., "Clinical uses of intravenous immunoglobulin," *Clinical & Experimental Immunology* 142, n. 1 (October 2005): 1-11. www.ncbi.nlm.nih.gov/pmc/articles/PMC1809480/ (accessed April 4, 2019).

4

A FUNCTIONAL APPROACH TO NEUROLOGICAL HEALTH

by Melanie Alarcio, M.D.

MY NAME IS MELANIE ALARCIO, and I'm a pediatric neurologist. I am a foreign medical graduate—I graduated from a medical school in the Philippines and did my initial pediatric residency there, specializing in neonatal intensive care. Then, I had my degree but needed to do another residency if I wanted to be a doctor here in the United States. I decided to do a fellowship in neurology. At Children's Hospital in Los Angeles, I was exposed to a lot of autoimmune neurologic disorders because the program director there was the foremost author and researcher on something called Opsoclonus myoclonus, which is an autoimmune disorder. I got exposed to many autoimmune disorders, and learned that a lot of them were Strep related.

I finished my fellowship and moved to Arizona, where I was hired by Phoenix Children's Hospital. All my patients who came to me with tic disorders, I would just ask: "How much of this is Strep related?"

I started attending conferences and began realizing the immune system and the brain are not disconnected; the brain's not isolated. I became interested in the gut microbiome (this was over ten years ago, before people had started talking about a healthy gut). When I would give antibiotics to my patients to treat PANS or PANDAS, I would automatically give them a probiotic, and they would get better. The gut got better as well.

I started getting more patients—not just PANS and PANDAS patients, but things like NMDA receptor antibody patients and other auto-antibody or immune-related patients as well.

As a result, I started attending more conferences. One of those, of which now I am a fellow, is called Medical Academy of Pediatric Special Needs. This organization is an offshoot of Autism Spectrum Disorder (ASD) research. A lot of research has been pointing to autism being an immune-related disorder in some patients. I got exposed to patients whose autism symptoms would resolve, as in totally disappear, after treating immune deficiencies. They wouldn't even fit the diagnostic criteria.

I kept practicing and attending conferences that took a more integrative approach to treatment. I got injured by a patient at Phoenix Children's Hospital, so I left and started working in private practice. It was mostly an adult neurology practice. I had a little leeway in what I could do, but I couldn't do all the biomedical and functional/integrative treatments that I wanted to do. Fortunately, I was recently able to open my own practice.

The Time to Ask Why

Western medicine is great. The problem is, here in the U.S., medicine is primarily symptom-based. You have a headache? Here is a drug for it. What happened to, "Why do you have a headache?"

Nobody asks why, and that's too bad. A patient may be coming to me for chronic migraine, for example, and it turns out their vitamin D is very low, or they have thyroid problems, or iron deficiency problems. Address *those*. Similarly, when a child's behavior suddenly changes, the thinking is generally, oh my God, he's ADHD! The standard course of action is to go see the psychiatrist and get a drug. I don't have anything against the drugs, because those drugs have a place. But I think what is lacking in Western medicine is the time to look at the underlying process. Patients are seen 15 minutes at a time. That's why I cannot be a hospital-employed doctor. They would fire me in two weeks because I take my time with a patient. I need the timeline; I try to figure out, *when* did *what* go wrong? When was your last normal?

My role is to find out: is there something underlying all of this? A lot of times, I find it. Sometimes, I don't. New things keep on coming out as I dig, and I continue to find answers. We have all these lab tests available, all this imagining, yet nobody wants to use them. This bothers me, because it's not as if we're living in the 17th century. At that time, when you practiced medicine, you looked, you touched, and based on what you saw and the list of symptoms, you made your best guess. You didn't have labs, you couldn't see under a microscope. But we *have* all those tools now. So, why aren't people using them? Why aren't doctors using them?

To me, patients need to be aware that doctors should be looking at *all* of them, not just part of them. So, for example, if you have a GI problem, you have diarrhea and constipation, the question is why? Are you not eating enough fiber? Or do you have parasites? People should ask the why.

There are labs now that will do a nasal culture and tell you what bacteria, or virals, or fungals are growing. If they do a sensitivity test, they'll know what antibiotic those bugs are sensitive to. But, generally speaking, most doctors won't do that because it takes time for the culture to come back, and we need to treat the patient that same day, using the listing of symptoms. The choice of antibiotics is trial and error because there is no way of knowing in the moment, using a rapid Strep test, if the bug you have will be sensitive to a particular antibiotic. One of the things the doctor can do is follow the patients closely. But again, it's not something that every doctor can do.

The Blood-Brain Barrier

They used to think that the blood-brain barrier protects everything, that it isolates the brain. But the weakest link of this barrier is in the hypothalamus because it's only a single-cell layer. And your hypothalamus sits above your sinuses, which is part of your respiratory tract. The olfactory endings, the nerve endings in your nose, they actually go straight into the olfactory cortex right beneath the hypothalamus, and there's no barrier at all. Toxins, inflammatory proteins, bacteria, microbes can go directly to the brain.

The blood-brain barrier is very reactive and aware of the environment, your body. There are really no immune cells in your brain but the glial cells, which are support cells in your brain, can transform and become immune-mediated, antigen-presenting cells. That's when you have molecular mimicry and they start attacking your own brain cells.

Molecular mimicry is the most common way that a bacterial or viral infection can trigger an autoimmune disorder. You have bacteria that triggers antigen changes or glial changes in your brain. Because whatever happens in your body, your brain finds out about it, especially in terms of what's happening in the gut. Seventy percent of your immune system is in your gut. And so, through the Vagus nerve, which connects your gut and your brain, you can get the glial changes that start attacking brain receptors. It's an immune-mediated response that causes cellular inflammation. It's like a cell danger response that leads to tic behaviors.

Genetic Testing

There are a lot of genetic testing technologies that are coming out. Parents, if they have children who have immune problems, should talk to their providers and ask, "Hey, can we run genetics testing on this?" Make sure the insurance will cover the testing. Again, we're not living in the 17th century. Insurance and treatment need to catch up. Right now, I have a hard time getting MTHFR genetic mutation testing covered, getting the HLA (human leukocyte antigen) test covered. Fortunately, it's not that expensive if you do have to pay out-of-pocket.

Some of the consumer genetics tests are useful, like the 23andme test. I have patients who use them when they go on sale for $59 or $99, and it gives us certain information—not the complete picture—and but it does provide some information to use when insurance won't cover genetics testing. Doctors can run the results through software that's been developed by specialists.

Boosting Our Immune Systems

Our immune system is adaptive, it adapts to our environment. Right now, everything in the world is toxic. There's not a single square inch that hasn't been exposed. It's in our soil, it's in our water, it's in our air. Electromagnetic frequencies are all around us, we're just being bombarded. So, a good diet helps cellular signaling. We really need to boost our immune systems to try help them detox all of things that we are exposed to. We have to help our immune system remain functioning. If you are on antibiotics, a probiotic supplement is a good idea. If you know your diet is all junk food, then yes, you may need a supplement. Again, it's the basics. Get a varied diet.

As far as what age it is safe to use supplements, there is no one answer. For example, you have baby probiotics. These are especially good for those born via C-section not exposed to vaginal flora, which is a baby's first introduction. That's what colonizes a baby's gut. So, this is why some babies get probiotics, to start helping their immune system to develop.

Omega-3, I can give at two years old. These fatty acids help with the development of the cell membranes in your brain. Plus, omega-3 is a very good anti-inflammatory.

Most of us do not get enough sun, so vitamin D may be needed.

One thing to be aware of is most vitamins contain folic acid, but folic acid cannot be metabolized. It has to be in the folate form so that the bacteria in our gut can metabolize it and it can be absorbed. There's a place for vitamins and minerals and supplements. I tend to use them specifically to address certain things, but eating a healthy diet—fruits, vegetables, meats, breads—really *balancing* what you're eating can lead to better health.

Keep Asking Why

Neurologists don't have the time to take an extensive medical history from patients. In medical school, everyone is taught about the importance of history and physical exam first, but the reality is there's no time. You focus on the symptom. So, I don't know where this is headed. The bigger centers like Duke, Stanford, Georgetown, Mayo, even at the University of Arizona and Banner, they have Autoimmune Encephalitis centers. But is it a comprehensive approach? I don't know.

For me, it's personal. I'm treating *you*, the person. Not your symptoms, not your labs. That's how I was trained—look at the person, not his numbers. Western doctors need to be more open to an integrative approach.

Ask the why. Look for answers. Keep asking why.

5

THE ROLE OF DIET

I WAS WILLING TO TRY anything when our son got so sick. We became more educated on the role of diet in gut health and worked to do whatever we could to bolster our son's compromised immune system. As a result, we cut out gluten and restricted sugar for two years. You'll read more about the reasoning behind this step in Dr. Appleton's section of the book in Chapter 7. Now, we have allowed casein back in our son's diet and mild amounts of gluten and sugar. Making these changes was more work for me, but has been good for our family overall as we cook more "whole food" dinners rather than grabbing something quick at a restaurant or consuming something premade by someone else out of the pantry or freezer.

We ended up severely limiting dairy for only about three to six months, just enough to get our son's body to calm down. It was overreacting. When you have an autoimmune response in multiple ways, it's your body saying, "Hey!" Today, we eat a lot of cheese in our house. You often hear people talking about anti-inflammatory foods, but it's like, "Well, why don't we talk more about what's *causing* the inflammation in the first place?"

The gluten we cut out totally for a good year, year and a half. When we're out and about today, we don't necessarily restrict gluten. But when we're home, I try and use gluten-free bread if I'm making sandwiches. We make a conscious decision to keep our house as gluten-free as possible. I just think, in general, we're eating way too much bread in this country. It's on and in everything. If we can limit ourselves to once a day, that will make an impact.

The Importance of Our Children's Gut Flora

According to researchers, the intestinal microflora is a positive health asset that critically influences the normal structural and functional development of the immune system.[45] Manipulation of the flora by consuming certain foods, beverages and/or supplements to enhance the beneficial components of our kids' gut microbiome could be a promising therapeutic strategy—and may even prevent health problems in the first place.

According to research, the flora in our digestive tract has a metabolic activity equal to an organ within an organ. The mechanisms guiding the influence of the bacteria on immune responses are beginning to be more understood. Therefore, an improved understanding of our gut flora will help us improve human health and ultimately reduce infectious, inflammatory and neoplastic disease processes.[46]

---

45 O'Hara, AM, "The gut flora as a forgotten organ," *EMBO Reports* 7, n.7 (July 2006): 688-693. www.ncbi.nlm.nih.gov/pmc/articles/PMC1500832/ (accessed April 3, 2019).

46 O'Hara, AM, "The gut flora as a forgotten organ," *EMBO Reports* 7, n.7 (July 2006): 688-693. www.ncbi.nlm.nih.gov/pmc/articles/PMC1500832/ (accessed April 3, 2019).

It can be challenging to think about our kids' microbiome, or gut flora, when we're attending to a thousand other family details. A lot of times—and I was guilty of this—our children want something like carbohydrate-heavy macaroni and cheese, chicken fingers, things that are easy to eat, and we give it to them. These easy foods taste good; they're salty, sugary snacks.

The problem is, of course, there aren't a lot of nutrients in these types of grab-and-go foods to create a nice foundation for these kids when they come into contact with bacteria and viruses. (And they *will* come into contact with bacteria and viruses. We can't keep our kids in a bubble.)

It's how my kids ended up with ear infections and sinus infections. One of my kids had to have tubes in his ears, and I think back to all of the stuff I should have done differently. I think back to my other son who was constipated a lot. If I had forced him to eat more fruits and vegetables or given him a probiotic, rather than giving him MiraLAX (which is what the doctor told me to do), it would have been so much better for his system than stripping out the good and the bad gut flora.

There are so many things we could or should do differently, as parents, to help our kids' bodies heal from the inside out, instead of just giving them a pill or a chemical that treats a symptom.

If I had it to do over again, I would've offered my children a wider array of fruits and vegetables from an earlier age. I don't think we should be afraid to send our children to bed complaining that they didn't get their chicken fingers. For me, I was always afraid of that temper tantrum. As you get older, you get more and more used to these tantrums. Now, it's about playdates and driving. But when you're a first-time mother or a tired mother, it's like, "Okay, fine. Whatever. Have the chicken fingers."

I'm excited that there are more natural food options now that are easy for parents to grab. That wasn't always the case.

Kari's Journey and Success Story

Eleven years ago, in the spring of my son's kindergarten year, he started to experience facial tics. His doctor attributed it to allergies and said, "Don't worry about it, he'll be fine." It went on all during the following summer. I had a friend who mentioned PANDAS at that time [editor's note: today, PANDAS is often diagnosed under the umbrella of Autoimmune Encephalopathy]. This friend said she'd heard it was caused by a Strep infection. I didn't think my son had ever *had* Strep. But I did call the doctor and ask for a culture, just to see. It was negative. At that time, I didn't know that Strep can be anywhere in your body. I didn't know you needed to do a blood test to find it.

On September 16, 2008, my son started saying the word 'damn,' uncontrollably, thousands of times a day. He also began having motor tics, first simple and then complex. His personality changed and he was screaming, "Mommy make it stop, my brain is making me do this, make it stop!" Our pediatrician sent us first to a child psychiatrist. Because I had heard of PANDAS, I kept saying to him, "Do you think this is what it could be?" He said it didn't exist, it wasn't real. He prescribed medication for Tourette's and said that *I* needed mental health services to learn to accept my child. While it took a long time before I actually stopped going to this psychiatrist, I knew right then it wasn't a fit. I eventually fired him. Meanwhile, Alex developed more symptoms, including sensitivity to light and sound, anxiety and stomach aches. It's like we were losing him, cognitively, physically and emotionally.[47]

As we desperately searched for answers, we met more and more doctors. My son has had a total of 26 doctors in five states and two countries.

It took us two and a half years to get the PANDAS diagnosis. My son went for *two and half years* with a misdiagnosis of Tourette's Syndrome. Every doctor who saw him said that he was the worst case of "Tourette's they had ever seen. We had our pediatrician, at one point, telling me to take him to Cincinnati to a doctor who could have a grid implanted in his brain. That's how bad it was.

The Root Cause

Because I taught child development and brain research for years before, I believed there had to be a root cause of what was happening. A few months after our initial visit to our pediatrician in 2008, my son was cultured again, but at that time, the doctor ordered a blood test as well. He called me back and said, "The blood test for Strep was positive."

I kept saying, "What's the root cause?" People don't just flip out, unless there is a reason. We went to a pediatrician in Chicago who is a leading expert in PANDAS. He's connected to the National Institute of Mental Health with Dr. Susan Swedo,

---

47 Vicki Louk Balint, "PANDAS: My brain is making me do this!" *Raising Arizona Kids* (July 1, 2012) www.raisingarizonakids. com/2012/07/pandas-my-brain-is-making-me-do-this/ (accessed April 10, 2019).

the person who identified this disorder in the first place. It wasn't until I got my son to him that we received a true diagnosis.

Inflammation—and that's what Autoimmune Encephalitis essentially is—was a huge factor in my son's behaviors. Years after the initial onset, we had one of his inflammation markers tested, and his number was 18,000. Normal was between 800 and 2300, so he was nine or ten times above normal. I showed one of our doctors, Amy Derksen, N.D., some video clips of his symptoms before he had any treatment, and she said, "Oh, I have kids like that now. My guess is his levels were between 40,000 and 50,000 when symptoms were at their worst." This would be twenty times above normal.

Turning Points

In addition to getting the right diagnosis and connecting with the right doctors, there were many game-changers in terms of bringing my son back to health. Getting his tonsils out was one of them. Had I known, I would've had it done sooner. He had his tonsils out between his second and third IVIG treatments (he's had five). What we now know is that they were hard as rocks when the doctor took them out. They looked okay, but they were smaller than normal and the doctor said he believed it was from years of fighting infection. We had requested they be cultured, and that never happened. So, I don't know what was in them. But many people find out, after having their tonsils removed, that there is a lot of infection in them and that's why they weren't getting better.

Nutrition was a big turning point for us. It's not as much as a player right now because he's so much better, but for about two years we were gluten free, casein free. We ate as many whole foods and organic foods as possible, foods that were minimally processed. However, this is largely how we ate before. Sugar was, and still is, a known trigger. A small amount of sugar, even occurring naturally in fruit, could set off my son's tics. Another thing to look at is glyphosate, an herbicide used on grains to regulate plant growth and regulate crops.[48] I'm not an expert on this, so do your own research, but I've read there are a lot of people who can't eat gluten in this country because of our use of this chemical.

When our son was in middle school, we were very strict about diet and sleep because I knew that when he became overtired, we would see an increase in his tics pretty quickly. I had a parent call me one time, a parent I felt was a friend. Not many people knew what we were going through because I didn't really talk about it, other than to family. Anyway, she said some of the other parents had been talking and wanted to tell me to lighten up on my son, to stop being so strict with him about his diet and sleep habits. It was shocking to me that another parent took it upon herself to tell me how to raise my child without having a clue of what we were dealing with medically.

It was very difficult, but I decided to take what she was saying not as a criticism, although my blood was starting to boil, but from a perspective of caring. I chose to see her as a person who cared and who had good intentions, so I shared a few details of what we had been going through. By the time I finished, and I didn't talk for more than four or five minutes, she was like, "Oh,

---

48 Glyphosate General Fact Sheet, *National Pesticide Information Center* npic.orst.edu/factsheets/glyphogen.html (accessed April 10, 2019).

I had no idea." No one knows what's really going on with your family unless you tell them.

That day, my son started to become more of an adult. I showed his blood work lab results to him and helped him to understand exactly how what he put into his body affected those numbers. I told him it was *his* turn to be in charge, that I would help him, but that he was old enough to make decisions and take responsibility for his own health—to stay well through nutrition, through supplements, and by getting enough sleep.

Homeopathy has also helped in getting my son to where he is now. Homeopathy is a medical system developed in the late 1700s in Germany. This natural approach to healing is based on an understanding that *like cures like*. Homeopathy is also based on the belief that the body can cure itself. Those who practice it use tiny amounts of natural substances, like plants and minerals, to stimulate the healing process.[49] This approach is non-invasive and there are no side effects. It works at the level of energy. If you would've told me this ten years ago, I would've said, "Sure, and I bet Cocoa Puffs work, too." I didn't know about it; I didn't understand. I think, to a person who hasn't gone through what I've gone through, they would look at this sort of thing and think you're a little cuckoo. But when you've tried everything else and exhausted every other option, you look for whatever is left. And that's what we did … and it worked!

We've done everything. I tried not to do everything at once; I tried to be a scientist, to not to change more than one variable at a time so I could see if things were getting better or if things were getting worse.

---

49 "What is Homeopathy?" WebMD www.webmd.com/balance/what-is-homeopathy (accessed April 10, 2019).

Spreading Knowledge

In those early years, there was nothing online. There was no support group. I helped start support groups; I was the Arizona co-leader for seven years and the national coordinator for support groups via PANDASnetwork.org. We were able to greatly increase the number of support groups around the country. I also fielded calls from desperate parents 24/7 for years. There were others who helped with the support groups as well at this time.

I was a part of the creation of a foundation that led to the founding of the first center of excellence in the world, in Tucson, with the National Institute of Mental Health, the University of Arizona Medical Center, and Banner Hospitals. There were people who were treating PANDAS before, but this is the first place that's doing the diagnosis, the treatment, and training in the medical school. They're training the doctors and doing research; they're doing all of it. Banner wants to expand to the other six states where they have a presence. I don't know the timeline, but this has definitely taken on a life of its own.

The motto for PANDASnetwork.org is "Know the symptoms, change the outcome."[50] My advice for anyone going through this now is don't ever stop. Always believe that your child can get better. What do I wish I had known 12 years ago? Get a Strep test—and not just a culture, get a blood test and don't stop treating the Strep until you test and retest to make sure it's gone.

It's not just the illness that you're fighting. You're fighting doctors who don't understand, although we don't have that as much now. But when we were going through this, there were

---

50 http://pandasnetwork.org/ (accessed April 10, 2019).

only five doctors that I knew of in the world who were able to diagnose it. Today, they're teaching it at medical schools.

It's fighting insurance companies. It's dealing with parents who don't understand. It's dealing with friends who don't understand why you're so depleted emotionally. A lot of PANDAS kids can hold it together at school, so people think it's not so bad. But then they come home and kind of implode.

There were a couple of times we had to take our son to the emergency room because his motor tics were so bad, we weren't sure if he was having a seizure or not. I would tell the doctors what was going on, but they'd never heard of PANDAS. They said, "What do you want us to do?" *They* were asking *me*.

Today, my son is approximately 95% better, 95% of the time.

This isn't a journey I asked for, it's not something I would want for any family. But the important thing is we are making progress and getting the right answers to the people who need them today. My message is this: If a doctor tells you your child won't heal, move on. Find a new doctor. I learned this the hard way. One of my promises to God is to share as much as I can about what I have learned to stop other families from having to go through what we did.

6

LIFESTYLE CHANGES

WHEN OUR SON WAS SO sick, I had people asking me, "Pam, why aren't you taking off work? Why aren't you home-schooling him?"

The practical matter of it was, A) we needed the income to pay for the doctor bills, and B) they said that he might have this forever, so my thinking was that our son might as well get used to being a productive citizen, because I couldn't afford to take care of him for the rest of my life. In other words, it just wasn't practical for me to end my career and become a full-time care-giver. Most parents are in the same boat as we were.

I thought, "This kid is going to have to learn to be a fighter." I even talked like that. I said, "I'm sorry that you have a headache today and I know that this is miserable, but just get through the day and learn at school and we'll cuddle tonight."

I did find someone on Care.com and we still use that person from 3 to 5 PM. That's the hardest period of time for me as a working mother. While my husband and I are still working, the kids need to get home, have their snacks, and get started on their homework.

Adjusting Our Environment

In the wake of our son's illness, I really looked into trying to remove more chemicals from our home. Unfortunately, my analysis was that it's nearly impossible to get rid of all the toxins in our environment. The fact is, our immune systems are bombarded with toxins every day, which is why we need them to operate optimally.

Our family did end up moving so that our house is at least two miles away from a freeway. It's not in a landing zone of an airport, and it's at least a mile away from any power lines. We did do that, and that's probably kind of extreme, but there's a lot of studies about electromagnetism and the pollution that comes off of power lines. We pulled out the carpet from the house we moved into and put in tile to reduce the dust. Dust can create an inflammatory response and hold in toxins; carpet is supposed to put off toxins for 10-15 years.

I try to buy natural hand and dish soaps as well. We also have our son use Listerine before and after brushing his teeth. We have all started this protocol and both illness and allergies are much less frequent for everyone in our family. These are, environmentally, the changes that we made.

7

Q&A WITH IMMUNOLOGIST RYAN CASPER, M.D.

Can you share a bit about your background and encounters with children suffering from symptoms similar to those of Pam's son?

I have been a board-certified clinical immunologist for almost 12 years. I started seeing PANS patients [editor's note: PANS is now generally being diagnosed under the Autoimmune Encephalopathy (AE) umbrella] early in my career, when Dr. Chris Spiekerman and I realized that we were seeing many kids with similar symptoms, including acute onset OCD tendencies, enuresis, tantrums, tics/strange movements, etc. Many of these symptoms were occurring immediately after Strep throat or other illnesses. We both knew about PANS but we had always been skeptical that it really existed. When we got together and talked in 2008 or 2009, we realized that there was really something to the diagnosis.

Pam and other parents of kids with autoimmune problems often face incorrect diagnoses for their children. Many parents are told, for example, that their kids need psychoactive drugs to treat tics and other behavioral symptoms. Where are we today in terms of mainstream Western medicine and AE understanding? What is the current healthcare status quo regarding autoimmune issues?

I think, unfortunately, we still have a lot of pediatricians who are unfamiliar with or uneducated about PANS. I was taught in residency (early 2000s) that PANS was a sham diagnosis and didn't really exist. I think a lot of primary doctors still hold that belief. However, it has gained some traction in the academic world of pediatrics, namely places like NIH and Stanford. There are now practice parameters on how to diagnose and treat PANS which gives more credibility to the diagnosis. But…I hear the phrase "My pediatrician doesn't believe in PANS" at least once a month.

Can you explain how a bacterial or viral infection can "trigger" autoimmune disease in children?

That's pretty tough to answer in a paragraph and, to be honest, it is not completely understood. Essentially, the autoimmune complications of PANS are caused by an atypical immune response to antigens (foreign proteins) of Strep bacteria that cross-react with self tissues and self proteins. So, the patient's immune system is basically "overreacting" to the Strep infection and starts attacking its own cells in the brain. Younger children (1 to 12 years) are more susceptible to PANS because they have more frequent Strep exposure and typically respond to infections with a more robust immune response than older adolescents and adults.

What are your thoughts on antibiotics as a tool for treating autoimmune issues in kids? Is there such a thing as too much?

I wouldn't recommend treating most autoimmune diseases with antibiotics. For instance, we do not treat lupus with antibiotics. Antibiotic therapy does not decrease immune responses in patients. The reason antibiotic therapy might work for PANS is that it rids the patient of chronic Strep infection (or possibly skin/sinus infections), which, in turn, decreases the autoimmune response. I do not like to use chronic antibiotic therapy as a treatment for PANS because there is risk for antibiotic resistance and other complications like *C. difficile.*

What do you wish more parents understood about nutrition and immune health?

The biggest thing is how important a balanced diet is to promote good immune system health. There is also some data that certain vitamins can be helpful, including vitamin D. Antioxidants have also been proven useful, as have zinc and quercetin. Some herbs also have been shown to have immune augmenting effects in some studies, including turmeric. Certainly, probiotics have clearly been shown to boost immune function in most patients.

8

HOMEODYNAMIC BALANCE: A Q&A WITH JEREMY APPLETON, N.D.

Can you speak to the divide between conventional and alternative medicine approaches to complex health conditions?

There are many conditions, particularly those classified as autoimmune, where conventional medicine falls short, in part because it sometimes lacks a holistic, integrated systems approach. Conventional medicine as it is practiced today has regrettably lost sight of the whole person, and instead aims to treat specific mechanistic problems with targeted drug therapies. Sometimes this is just what a person needs, but for baffling autoimmune conditions, this is rarely the case. "Here is your diagnosis. We understand the mechanism of that to be X and we have this a drug that interrupts that mechanism. Here is a prescription." Often this produces relief of symptoms, perhaps dramatically so, but it may fail miserably at addressing the root cause of the disorder. Or side effects of the drug could mask or worsen the problem in the long term, even as they relieve symptoms.

Consider a bacterial infection. Antibiotics can kill a bacterium, and in many cases, this is a cure for the disease. But antibiotics can have unintended effects, like killing good gut bacteria along with the bad, disrupting the balance of organisms that make up our microbiome. We now know it is very important that people have good bacteria in their gut.

Can diet and lifestyle make a difference in chronic and complex health conditions?

One big obstacle to overall health is the way people eat. Diet contributes to the development of chronic disease, and may also be a factor in cases of unexplained disease. If the body is adversely reacting, sometimes chronically, to the habitual ways in which we are eating, it can be enormously helpful to break the pattern, to clear the playing field. It is well documented, for example, that simple fasting can dramatically improve symptoms and inflammation, as in rheumatoid arthritis. I have found that an elimination-reintroduction diet can also be quite useful in resolving symptoms, while at the same time being the gold standard—more than any lab test—for identifying potential dietary triggers.

Food and diet are so important that everyone seems to have an opinion about them. We all have to feed ourselves every day, multiple times a day. And so, food is a topic that interests most people. It obsesses some people, from gourmands to health food enthusiasts, and it is subject to fads.

Food and food production have changed; grains aren't what they once were, and neither are our immune systems. Some people legitimately can't digest gluten well, even if they don't have celiac disease. But then it becomes faddish, and too many people say "Oh, I have to eliminate gluten." Not necessarily. Listen to your body. Do an elimination-reintroduction diet. Find out; there is wisdom within.

Identifying the components in a person's diet that may be problematic is a powerful tool, and removing offending food-stuffs while replacing them with more nourishing options be life-transforming. Remove obstacles to cure; food may be one of them. The foods we crave the most are, ironically, sometimes the most problematic ones.

How does diet affect those with autoimmune diseases?

For people with autoimmune diseases or other unexplained health challenges, one size does not fit all in terms of treatment or lifestyle changes. There are all kinds of investigations and test-ing that one can potentially do to identify what the exacerbating factors for the disease might be. Functional medicine offers many diagnostic tools. But sometimes the simplest changes yield the most dramatic results. They may be the hardest to accomplish, at least at first, but worth the effort. And once you start feeling better, you gain momentum and motivation to keep going. Like exercise.

Kids are notorious about the kinds of diets they prefer to eat. Kids, even more than adults, love sugar. They *love it*. Sugar is yummy, and sugar's a treat, and kids can get really out of bal-ance in their diet. It sure is hard to get a kid to eat less sugar; they are wired for it even more than adults. But oftentimes, if one has an autoimmune condition, sugar can have adverse ef-fects. It adversely alters the gut microbiome. It alters how we metabolize nutrients. It alters brain activity. It can exacerbate a candida infection if one happens to be present. Sugar can throw us off balance in many different ways. It can depress the immune system's ability to fight an infection. Taking a break from sugar is hard at first, but notice how it makes you feel.

Alternative and Functional Medicine seem very complicated. There are so many moving parts; how do I know what's actually working?

When you take a multifactorial approach to healing—including diet, lifestyle, environment, supportive natural medicines, etc.—you won't necessarily know *exactly* what worked. That's why some mainstream doctors get skeptical about multi-modal, natural medicine because they don't know what worked, and they don't know how to test for what worked. It's not a magic bullet or a single drug that you can test in a double-blind clinical study. They might throw their hands up and say, "I don't know. Whatever you were doing, just keep doing it," or they just write it off as placebo effect.

It is also challenging because many practitioners in the so-called "alternative medicine" space are neither skilled nor ethical, and there are indeed a lot of scams out there. So how does one tell the difference between legitimate, albeit unproven, alternatives to conventional medicine, and outright quackery? It takes persistence and self-education and talking to many people, learning many perspectives.

So-called "alternative" or "integrative" or "functional" medicine can be difficult to study using conventional medical models because the conventional medical model wants a mono-therapy.

That's the way you do it, the double-blind study. Half the people—they don't know which half—get a single intervention, and the other half don't, and during the study, the doctors and the patients are all "blinded" so we can rule out the placebo effect because the mind is indeed a powerful healer.

But if somebody's got a complex health problem or an environmental sensitivity and they're using natural medicine, they're not going to try just one single intervention: "Okay, I'll just take turmeric." Who's got time for that? Anyway, it's less likely to work than if it was taken in the context of other beneficial changes. The desperate parent who has a sick kid is going to use everything in their toolbox that might help their child. Wouldn't you?

Then improvements start happening. Was it the diet? Was it the removal of a toxin or allergen in the environment? Was it the probiotic, which helped improve the intestinal microbiome, and thus immune function? Was it the anti-inflammatory? Was it the adaptogen that helped with the hypothalamic-pituitary-adrenal (HPA) axis? Was it the fact that the kid is sleeping better and the immune system was able to finally catch up? Is it nutrients improving mitochondrial dysfunction? Or more nutritious food correcting a longstanding deficiency? Is it less pesticide residue exposure in the food because of eating more "organic?" Or is it some blend of several or all of those things? More likely some combination. The body's systems are all interconnected, one affects the other. This is why holistic approaches to healing can be so effective when conventional mono-therapies fail.

How do you choose an approach when a condition is of unknown origin?

The way that you approach an unexplained or complex disease condition, as many autoimmune diseases are, is by treating the whole person, not just the "disease". We don't know what causes autism, so we treat the child. We look to what is known in the research and we go from there, and start weaving together the threads of evidence that we have. We may see that autistic kids have mitochondrial dysfunction, or their neurotransmitters like serotonin are dysregulated. Or they have problems in their gut microbiome. And then we look for the connections between the systems. But often we find that if you start with the gut, heal the gut first, many other problems will resolve, even when they appear distant to or unrelated to digestion or intestinal function. The Greek physician Hippocrates famously said, "All disease begins in the gut." There is wisdom in this. When in doubt, it is a good place to start.

The holistic physician, the naturopathic doctor, the integrative medical doctor, they often are searching for unifying explanations that could harmonize the story of an illness. So, they take what's called a functional medicine approach, a systems approach. They ask, "How do we optimize these complex and interacting systems?" The gut microbiome, the HPA axis of the endocrine system, the neurobiological mechanisms of neurotransmitters, and inflammatory mediators of the immune system. In the body, those systems are all interacting with each other anyway; you can't just touch one of them without sending ripples through the others. The more integrative approaches take advantage of this interconnectedness, accomplishing multiple clinical objectives at once.

How can treating the gut help with a condition of the brain?

The gut and the brain are intimately connected, through the actual wiring (the Vagus nerve, notably); through neurotransmitters and neurotransmitter-like substances originating in the gut; through our gut microbiome's close interaction with our immune systems (in the gut-associated lymphoid tissue); in the endocrine system, and the various hormones it produces; and in the substances that can leak across the gut barrier into the bloodstream and affect mood, cognition and behavior. Collectively, these pathways of bi-directional communication are known as the Gut-Brain Axis. An explosion of research over the last 10 years has been elucidating these pathways, and in particular the contribution of the gut microbiota, the bacteria that live in our intestines, and their direct effects on our neurological system—on mood, cognition, even neuromuscular function—via these pathways.

For example, gut bacteria ferment fiber we cannot digest and produce short-chain fatty acids, such as propionic acid, butyric acid and the like. Short-chain fatty acids are used as fuel for the cells that line our intestines, our enterocytes. So, the bacteria have evolved to produce something of value to us, something that literally shapes the surface on which they reside. But short chain fatty acids are far more than just fuel for intestinal cells. They can travel through the bloodstream to distant sites and act like neurotransmitters, act like serotonin or GABA or other neurotransmitters, and they can also influence the body's own production of those same neurotransmitters. In the case of a gut dysbiosis, an imbalance of bacteria in the gut, there can be profound dysregulation of these neurotransmitters, with significant effects on brain function, mood, etc.

You may have heard the term "leaky gut" or "leaky gut syndrome." It refers to intestinal permeability defects. When you have dysbiosis, it can lead to a leaky gut. From there, you have leakage of these bacterial cell wall byproducts and other substances that can lead to chronic inflammation, and from there potentially to neurologic or neuropsychiatric symptoms. The systems are connected, and they are directly influenced by the quality of the gut microbiome.

So how do we treat people with autoimmune disease? When somebody's coming to you with a complex, inflammatory, unexplained condition; or with an autoimmune disease … treat the gut. Start there. It can't hurt. Heal that first, and you will find the other problems may improve surprisingly. Remove the obstacles to the body's own natural healing capacities: environmental toxins, allergens, the lousy foods that people eat, and replace that with nourishing alternatives, a clean home, a home that doesn't have mold floating around in the air, organic foods that don't have pesticide residues on them, organic eggs or dairy that don't have antibiotic residues in them that could be adversely altering the microbiome. Cumulatively, if you clean up the diet and you clean up the environment, and then you start giving a child some natural therapies that are supportive—natural anti-inflammatories, rebuild the gut microbiome, support for mitochondria, etc.—you can have wide-ranging benefits. If nothing else, it will be complementary to whatever primary therapy is being used.

My medical doctor doesn't seem to have the time to get into all this with me.

Doctors are frustrated. They're frustrated because the way the medical system is set up; they only have six minutes to spend with a patient, or 12 minutes, or whatever. How are you going to get a comprehensive history of someone's diet and environmental exposures, their mental and emotional life? The little nuances that often hold clues to the underlying issues? It is impossible to get the whole story in just a few minutes, or even in a single extended visit.

We need physicians who are trained in a more holistic, systems paradigm of medicine, who can approach patients in a sophisticated, nuanced way. Unfortunately, many of the alternative practitioners operating outside of mainstream medicine are unscrupulous or inadequately trained. You get a lot of quackery mixed in with legitimate complementary medicine. When you have desperate people who are not well served by the system, they'll try anything. Sometimes they get preyed upon, or misled by unscrupulous charlatans. The persistent, self-educated ones who persevere will find their way to one of the many brilliant integrative healthcare practitioners out there, and for them, the results may be truly life-altering.

9

SUPPLEMENTS

WHEN OUR SON WAS SICK, I was really grasping at straws, and I was lucky enough to find Dr. Alarcio in Arizona. Next, I found an Italian man in a confidential Facebook group who said that in Europe, they healed many diseases with essential oils.

In college, I lived in London with three girls from Italy, and we stay in touch. So, I reached out to them and said, "Hey, do you know about essential oils? I'm told this can help my son." They said, "We don't know what that word is, but it could be a translation thing. Can you explain what you're talking about?" The pessimistic part of me is like, "Oh gosh, the Italian guy is full of it." But I said, "Well, he's saying things like oregano helps bacteria, that all of these extracts help treat viruses and bacterial infections."

They replied, "Yes, everybody knows that!" I'm said, "No, everybody does NOT know that."

It's possible the earth gives us everything we need, we just don't know how to use it in a healthful way, or in a way that makes money, which is what our society is geared toward. This has been very helpful in terms of growth and prosperity but has perhaps killed off some old ways of doing things, some old generational knowledge, that can help everybody in terms of health and wellness.

The Evidence

The scientific evidence in favor of wider use of essential oils is piling up. Experts in healthcare and in the food industry know there is a need for antimicrobial substances that can slow or halt the growth of potentially pathogenic microorganisms, while not negatively impacting beneficial gastrointestinal tract microflora in the way that antibiotics do.

A recent in vitro study examined the potential of a selection of essential oils as agents to treat dysbiosis, a gastrointestinal disorder in which your gut flora is out of balance. Eight essential oils were examined. Doubling dilutions of the essential oils were tested against 12 species of intestinal bacteria, which represent the major genera found in the human gastrointestinal tract. Results showed that the essential oils they tested inhibited the growth of potential pathogens at concentrations that had no effect on the beneficial bacteria examined.[51]

Likewise, essential oils may be protective against ulcers. Turmeric and ginger are widely used as traditional medicine and food ingredients. In a 2015 study, researchers evaluated the gastroprotective activity of turmeric essential oil and ginger

---

51 JA Hawrelak et al., "Essential oils in the treatment of intestinal dysbiosis: A preliminary in vitro study," *Alternative Medicine Review* 14, n. 4 (December 2009) www.ncbi.nlm.nih.gov/pubmed/20030464 (accessed April 2, 2019).

essential oil in rats. Turmeric and ginger were evaluated for their anti-ulcer activity against ethanol-induced ulcers in male Wistar rats at different doses: 100, 500 and 1000 mg/kg body weight.

Turmeric and ginger essential oils inhibited ulcer by 84.7% and 85.1%, respectively, as seen from the ulcer index.[52] As you can see, the evidence that essential oils have real effects on the body is quite compelling.

Irritable bowel syndrome (IBS) is a common gastrointestinal disorder associated with overgrowth of unhelpful bacteria in the small intestine. This disorder may be treated with antibiotics, but again, there is the concern that widespread antibiotic use might lead to antibiotic resistance. Some herbal medicines have been shown to be beneficial, so researchers conducted a preliminary study in vitro to compare the antibacterial activity of the essential oils of culinary and medicinal herbs against the bacterium, *E. coli*. Extracts of coriander, lemon balm, and spearmint leaves were tested for their antibacterial activity in a disc diffusion assay. Study results showed that peppermint and coriander seed oils were more potent than the antibiotic rifaximin.[53]

Essential oils can also help with anxiety and sleep issues. For example, the effect of Silexan™, a patented active substance with an essential oil produced from Lavandula angustifolia flowers,

---

52 Liju VB, et al., "Gastroprotective activity of essential oils from turmeric and ginger," *Journal of Basic Clinical Physiology and Pharmacology* 16, n. 1 (January 2015). www.ncbi.nlm.nih.gov/pubmed/24756059 (accessed April 2, 2019).

53 Thompson A, et al. "Comparison of the antibacterial activity of essential oils and extracts of medicinal and culinary herbs to investigate potential new treatments for irritable bowel syndrome," *BMC Complementary and Alternative Medicine* 28, n. 13 (November 2013). www.ncbi.nlm.nih.gov/pubmed/24283351 (accessed April 3, 2019).

was investigated in patients with anxiety-related restlessness and disturbed sleep. The study confirmed the calming and anti-anxiety efficacy of this supplement.[54]

They regularly use essential oils as supplements in Europe and Australia. I was talking to someone about it recently and asked, "Why do you think it's so prevalent in these parts of the world?" They said it was because medicine is so expensive there that you try everything that you can naturally, first.

Starting and Stopping Allergy Shots

In early 2015, at the direction of an immunologist, we started allergy shots for our son. We continued to pull lab work every 3-4 months to monitor his vitamin and immune system levels.

In early 2016, we stopped the allergy shots and are happily maintaining our son's health and the entire families' health with the use of daily probiotic, B12, D3, complete omega (or krill) oil, a gluten-free home and low-sugar diet, and a regimen of daily essential oils.

We are in good company, as researchers learn more and more about the power of plant extracts in both healing and preventative care. Numerous studies, for example, have shown the antibacterial effects of tea tree oil. One recent study, for instance, compared the healing times of patients with wounds infected with *Staph*. It looked at conventional treatment alone and conventional treatment plus fumes of tea tree essential oil.

---

54 Kasper S, et al., "Efficacy of orally administered Silexan in patients with anxiety-related restlessness and disturbed sleep—A randomized, placebo-controlled trial" *European Neuropsychopharmacology* 25, n. 11 (November 2015) www.ncbi.nlm.nih.gov/pubmed/26293583 (accessed April 3, 2019).

The results showed a significantly decreased healing time in participants treated with tea tree oil.[55] Likewise, combinations of essential oils including lavender and cinnamon have been shown to kill E. coli.[56] These extracts may work by weakening the cell wall of resistant bacteria. They contain secondary metabolites that are capable of inhibiting or slowing the growth of bacteria, yeasts, and molds.[57]

Our Supplement Protocol

Here's what we gave my son in the wake of his illness:

- Olive Leaf Extract (especially as needed when a viral infection is present)
- QBC and Copaiba as needed for inflammation (as a natural alternative to Motrin)
- Daily B12 and D3 for immune support
- Daily Omega-3s
- Daily Prebiotic/Probiotic

---

55 Chin KB and Cordell B, "The effect of tea tree oil on wound healing using a dressing model," *Journal of Alternative & Complementary Medicine* 19, n.12 (December 2013). www.ncbi.nlm.nih.gov/pubmed/23848210 (accessed May 6, 2019).

56 Yap PS, et al. "Antibacterial Mode of Action of Cinnamomum verum Bark Essential Oil, Alone and in Combination with Piperacillin, Against a Multi-Drug-Resistant Escherichia coli Strain," *Journal of Microbiology and Biotechnology* 25, n.8 (August 2015) www.ncbi.nlm.nih.gov/pubmed/25381741 (accessed May 6, 2019).

57 Nazzaro F, et al. "Effect of Essential Oil on Pathogenic Bacteria," *Pharmaceuticals* 6, n.12 (Published online November 2013) 1451-1474. www.ncbi.nlm.nih.gov/pmc/articles/PMC3873673/ (accessed May 6, 2019).

- Daily l-methylfolate (different than folic acid) for Ryan's heterogenous MTHFR 6 and 12
- PS (Phosphatidylserine) as needed for sleep at night. This supplement has also shown success for those with ADD and Anxiety.

Essential Oil Protocol

Using essential oils brought our son back to 100%. We changed the protocol after the first year. Here is the protocol we used for the first 9-12 months after he got so sick:

- Performed an essential oil massage once a week.
- Diffused 3-4 drops nightly of thieves, thyme, frankincense, and lavender. However, any of the oils can be diffused.
- Took capsules every day with a meal. Recipe: three drops each of oregano, thyme, thieves, frankincense, lavender, and copaiba. If a child cannot take the capsule, apply to the bottom of the feet. You may see a flare-up of symptoms, which is a result of a detox reaction. The symptoms are always temporary. For maintenance, we give our son one capsule a day plus rubbing his feet at night with oregano, cinnamon, cloves, turmeric, frankincense, and myrrh. Our entire house followed this regimen and we had all had different positive reactions ranging from no allergies to increased focus, better mood, better sleep, etc.

After the first year, we no longer found it necessary to do the essential oil massage once a week but are diligent in diffusing and taking oils regularly.

Why Supplements are Necessary

I've had friends tell me, "Pam, this whole thing is ridiculous. Just get what you need from food." But it's my understanding that the right foods don't even have the same nutrients that they did fifty years ago. Our farmland is over-farmed, the pest control is so much stronger than it once was, so the toxicity is higher. So, you've got to be thinking about, "What am I taking in? What is organic? What is safe to be non-organic?"

A lot of the chemicals in our food supply will prevent you from absorbing your vitamins and minerals correctly. If you have high amounts of toxicity in some of the stuff that's coming into your system, it'll prevent you from having a healthy balance. Your body has to attack *that* and cannot fix *this*.

It's important to eat right, to reduce our carbohydrates, to eat lots of lean meats and fruits and vegetables but in absence of that, especially in children or people with autoimmune disorders, it's crucial to really make sure that you have additional support there to take care of our bodies. Thus, supplementation is smart.

Sadly, we have seen many others who did not follow our path and instead went down the road of continued antibiotics, Advil, and regular IVIG treatments that are better for short periods but not for longer ones.

Benefits of Supplements for the General Population

Again and again, studies show that the microbiota in our guts could activate the immune and central nervous system (CNS). Gut microorganisms can produce substances such as serotonin and gamma-aminobutyric acid, which act on the brain.

Preclinical research in rodents suggests that certain probiotics have antidepressant and anti-anxiety activities.[58]

We have all certain predispositions to something. And we will all encounter something in life that will act as a trigger to whatever that predisposition is. My child had a predisposition to an autoimmune disorder, and when he got hit with a bacterial infection and a virus at the same time, that was his trigger. There's now a very interesting study that says that people with Alzheimer's may have had some serious infections in their lives that acted as their trigger and have been very slowly evolving.[59]

It begs the question: if you can limit the number of bacterial and viral infections you come into contact with, or that your body reacts to, how much better off will you be? We come into contact with stuff all the time, but is your body strong enough to fight it off? Or does it make its way in? What is the collateral damage from an infection? If we can prevent some of that damage from happening, we should. It's similar to a vaccine—you don't get the mumps, the measles, etc. when you have it.

Is it possible that by taking some of these supplements, it's almost like you're vaccinating your body and making it stronger to fight against anything that could act as a trigger to your

---

58 Evrensel A and Ceylan ME, "The Gut-Brain Axis: The Missing Link in Depression," *Clinical Psychopharmacology and Neuroscience* 13(3) December 2015; 239-244. www.ncbi.nlm.nih.gov/pmc/articles/PMC4662178/ (accessed April 3, 2019).

59 Yong E, "Even More Evidence for the Link Between Alzheimer's and Herpes: Several new studies have rejuvenated a long-dismissed idea that links the common brain disease to the viral infections," *The Atlantic* (July 2018) www.theatlantic.com/science/archive/2018/07/herpes-viruses-alzheimers/564887/ (accessed April 15, 2019).

genetic predispositions? It all comes back to healing from the inside out.[60] Are you making your cells stronger? Or are they just going to start not acting properly?

Hello Health

To proactively address chronic inflammation, high doctor bills, allergies, and the long-term use of both over-the-counter and prescription drugs, I sought the assistance of immunologists, neurologists, and naturopaths to get to the root of our family's health problems. I wanted to create a supplement combining all the things my family was taking into just one or two pills—at the request of my son.

Created under doctor care (Dr. Alarcio and one of her natural doctor partners), these combinations of supplements are like nothing else available on the market. I spent years searching for a product like this, to no avail. Hello Health supplements support the immune system against inflammation, bacterial and viral infections. They contain natural ingredients known to break through mucus layers and biofilms to get to the root of infections.

Your cells are always replicating. Various cells replicate at different rates depending on where they are located in the body. If your body can replicate healthy cells, instead of unhealthy autoimmune cells, that is really important for your overall health.

---

60 Rodriguez T, "Essential Oils Might be the New Antibiotics," *The Atlantic* (January 2015) www.theatlantic.com/health/archive/2015/01/the-new-antibiotics-might-be-essential-oils/384247 (accessed May 6, 2019).

Hello Health supplements support the body against future infections and inflammation, and naturally cross the blood-brain barrier when conventional antibiotics and antibacterial/antiviral medicine are unable to do so. They are for those suffering from systemic inflammation, compromised immune systems, and autoimmune illnesses such as celiac, encephalopathy, eczema, arthritis, long-term illnesses such as heart disease and neurological disorders.

My goal in creating this product was to support the body instead of masking symptoms. The ingredients combat today's aggressive bacteria and viruses as well as what is more recently naturally missing in the food supply and western diets. I am currently looking for integrative health professionals and nutraceutical companies to partner with us to bring these products to a wider market.

Who Should Take Hello Health?

If you've got susceptibility to bacteria and viruses, it's helpful to get some of these key essential oils and prebiotics/probiotics into your system regularly. Everyone in my family takes the supplements I developed. My kids rarely get colds and allergies and have avoided serious illnesses since we started taking these supplements. My husband doesn't, either. I used to get sick every single time I flew somewhere, and I fly a lot so I was sick a lot.

Since taking the supplements, I've had people tell me I'm not aging. I still have grays coming in, but my skin looks good. There's something to be said about getting these helpful substances right into your system and to your cells, as opposed to putting these oils on your skin. These substances naturally dissipate within your system in a very short span of time, so a regular dose is helpful.

The Right Path

There's nothing like the supplements I've developed available. I've looked and I've looked; I've gone in natural food stores, on Google and Amazon and there's just not this kind of thing available in these combinations in these small doses. My youngest son said, "Mommy, can you please put this into a few things, because I'm sick and tired of taking all of this stuff." I said, "Hmm, I don't know." So, I started the journey.

I had one national doctor call me and say, "What you're doing is wrong. You're going to hurt your health and your son's health." That freaked me out enough that I had my son's kidneys tested. They came back perfectly fine, but when I took him to the local Children's Hospital, I was half expecting CPS to be called. Testing his kidneys was not new to us as the doctor had us test his kidneys about one year following constant antibiotic and Advil/Motrin use. At that time, the results showed some unusual signs and they asked us to regularly monitor his kidneys. So, the clean bill of health was just another indication to me that I was on the right path.

There are so many doctors out there who feel so strongly because they were educated in a particular way, but there's more and more research coming out every day. So, they may or may not be educated with the latest data. It's frustrating. In any case, here is what's in our two main Hello Health supplements:

Immune & Brain Balancing: Complete Prebiotic and Probiotic Immune Support Formula, Cognition, Mood, Digestion Health

1. Prebiotics – Prebiotics are a specialized plant fiber that beneficially nourishes the beneficial bacteria already in the intestines. Think of prebiotics as the roughage that gives good bacteria a place to flourish in your gut.

2. Probiotics – Probiotics hold the key not just to better health and a stronger immune system, but also to healing digestive issues, mental health illness, and neurological disorders. Overall health begins in the gut.

3. D3 – Vitamin D3 is a vitamin derived from 7-dehydrocholesterol; however, vitamin D3 acquires hormone-like actions when cholecalciferol (vitamin D3) is converted to 1,25-dihydroxy vitamin D3 (Calcitriol) by the liver and kidneys. As a hormone, Calcitriol controls phosphorus, calcium, and bone metabolism and neuromuscular function; inadequate levels of D3 has been linked to impaired immunity and cancer.

4. 5-Methylfolate – L-5-MTHF is the metabolically active natural form of folic acid, which is found in nature (certain whole, unfortified foods) and plays a role in DNA synthesis and repair. One in three Americans has a genetic variation (the MTHFR variation) that impairs their ability to properly utilize folic acid (also known as vitamin B9). Supplementation can make a truly dramatic difference in your health.

Immune & Brain Nourishing: Powerful Herbal Formulation with Omegas that Supports Daily Immunity, Heart, Attention and Eliminates Toxins

1. Omega 3 – Omega-3 fatty acids boost anti-inflammatory agents, lower risk of coronary heart disease and improve cholesterol numbers. There have also been promising results from studies looking at omega-3 for depression, and attention-deficit hyperactivity disorder (ADHD).

2. Proprietary Blend of Eight Herbs:

    a. The first two ingredients are powerful antimicrobials with antibacterial, antiviral, and antifungal properties.

    b. The third relieves chronic stress and anxiety, reduces pain and inflammation, and boosts immunity.

    c. The fourth ingredient has powerful antioxidant, antifungal, antiviral, anti-inflammatory, antiparasitic, expectorant, and antispasmodic properties.

    d. The fifth is used in many cultures for treating arthritis, yeast infections, colds, flu, and digestive problems.

    e. The sixth contains terpenes, which are hydrocarbons that can reduce pain, eliminate inflammation, protect against infection, heal the skin, prevent fungal growth, boost respiratory health, improve the health of the skin and hair, improve bladder control, speed healing, and lower blood pressure.

f. The seventh ingredient has been used for
    thousands of years as an anti-inflammatory
    treatment; it is also known for anti-allergic,
    antibacterial, antimicrobial, antifungal, anti-par-
    asitic, antiviral, and anti-worm properties.

g. The final ingredient is an antioxidant, antibacte-
    rial, antimicrobial, anti-inflammatory substance,
    and has immune-stimulating properties. Its
    phenolics protects LDL cholesterol from
    oxidation; this is attributed to its anti-in-
    flammatory effects.

3. Phosphatidylserine – Phosphatidylserine supplements
    are touted as a natural remedy for a variety of health
    conditions, including attention deficit-hyperactivity
    disorder (ADHD), Alzheimer's disease, anxiety, depres-
    sion, multiple sclerosis, and stress.

The Impact of Hello Health

Our family takes these supplements and has regular blood
draws. Doctors not only found that infections and deficiencies
were reduced, but our lab work also showed decreased immunoglobulin E and increased immunoglobulin G and IgM levels,
indicators of overall immune function.

Immunoglobulin G is also known as IgG. People with IgG
deficiency are more likely to get infections. Although researchers don't know what causes primary IgG deficiency, genetics
may play a role. A blood test that measures immunoglobulin

can diagnose this condition.[61] Selective IgM deficiency is characterized by substantially reduced or absent serum IgM with normal or increased concentrations of other immunoglobulins.[62] Immunoglobulin E is an indicator of inflammation and inflammatory response in the body.

For our family, naturally getting to the root of the problem and attacking the infections and raising vitamin, mineral, IgG and IgM levels took time. Fortunately, we steadily improved with the help of these supplements, and eventually base-lined at optimal levels.

After becoming educated and involved in a community of others with pediatric issues including Pediatric Autoimmune Neuropsychiatric Disorder (PANS), Pediatric Autoimmune Neuropsychiatric Disorders Associated with Streptococcal Infections (PANDAS), Lyme, and Encephalopathy, my family ended up restoring our health. By being aggressive in seeking a combination of non-traditional medicine and traditional medicine approaches, we have achieved overall total health. We have also reduced health-related time and expenses.

Disclaimer: Hello Health is not approved by the FDA. Ask your doctor or caregiver before taking any supplement. Optimal results are seen with decreased gluten and sugar diet. These supplements were created under doctor instruction and personal experience.

---

61 "What are IgG deficiencies?" Reviewed by Antoine Azar, M.D. www.hopkinsmedicine.org/healthlibrary/conditions/allergy_and_asthma/igg_deficiencies_134,109 (accessed March 29, 2019).

62 Gupta S and Gupta A, "Selective IgM Deficiency—An Underestimated Primary Immunodeficiency," *Frontiers in Immunology* 8 (published online September 2017). www.ncbi.nlm.nih.gov/pmc/articles/PMC5591887/ (accessed May 13, 2019),

CONCLUSION

WRITING THIS BOOK WAS IMPORTANT to me because I want to help other families. Through much trial and error, I've found a way to help my children remain healthy, and I simply cannot keep it to myself. As other parents of children who've fallen unexpectedly ill have said, I didn't ask for this path. My career is actually in Operations and Technology, and I would be completely happy to keep it there. But circumstances forced me to change my thinking regarding health and wellness, and I want to offer you what I've learned, and what I've created in Hello Health.

Every day brings new headlines about the ways in which our minds and bodies are one. I was just reading about how Lyme disease can induce explosive anger,[63] and about how hormonal shifts during menopause can affect women's mental health.[64] We are learning more every year about the connection between gut health, our immune system, and our mental health. Add to this

---

63 https://www.ncbi.nlm.nih.gov/pmc/articles/PMC5851570/ Accessed May 6, 2019.

64 https://www.mdedge.com/psychiatry/article/175738/depression/ psychiatric-considerations-menopause Accessed May 6, 2019.

all of the concerning news about antibiotic-resistant bacteria, and it becomes overwhelmingly clear we need new tools to get and stay well.

My hope is that your family will benefit from the latest research and tools outlined in this book, and reach out to me to learn more about changing the conversation.

Our bodies are absolutely remarkable in a million different ways—but they are not machines. We cannot expect them to function day in and day out for decades without giving them the nutrients and phytochemicals they need to fight off disease. It's time to approach our health—and the health of our children—comprehensively. Join us.

ABOUT THE AUTHOR

PAMELA WIRTH is an avid learner and has a desire to help others. She brings her experience in operations, technology, and marketing to health and wellness. Ms. Wirth's experience and attention to detail allows her to solve problems from the top down and the bottom up.

Outside of work, she enjoys yoga, hiking, cooking, spending time with her husband and two children, and attending their respective hockey events.

Finally, Pamela is the co-founder of Hello Health Nutrition LLC, which is committed to delivering products aimed at the cognitive and immune effects stemming from autoimmune illnesses.

Made in the
USA
Columbia, SC